T0077994

CONQUERING ERECTILE DYSFUNCTION

RECLAIMING YOUR SEXUAL LIFE

W. R. MILLS

authorHOUSE

AuthorHouse™
1663 Liberty Drive
Bloomington, IN 47403
www.authorhouse.com
Phone: 833-262-8899

Published by AuthorHouse 04/27/2022

ISBN: 978-1-6655-5831-0 (sc)
ISBN: 978-1-6655-5830-3 (e)

CONTENTS

INTRODUCTION

According to the Mayo Clinic, Erectile Dysfunction (ED) is the inability to get and keep an erection firm enough for sex.

Although there are many medical causes for ED, not all of them are medical problems. If you are experiencing the symptoms of ED, the very first thing you need to do is consult your doctor.

If there are medical issues causing your ED, these MUST be addressed first.

Self-diagnosis and treatment are never a good idea, as ED can be a symptom of something that is life threatening.

Always seek the advice of your medical care provider first.

Having said that, the solutions, practices, and exercises you find in this book will change your life.

I am going to take you on a journey that involves every part of your being. The journey will start with a strong foundation for you to build upon. You will make changes that will not only affect your sexual life, but you entire life.

I believe that down deep, everyone wants to change their reality. Use this book as a means of changing yours.

PART 1

BREATHING

This section will deal with the mechanics of proper breathing and the effect it will have on Conquering Your Erectile Dysfunction.

CHAPTER 1

WHY PROPER BREATHING IS IMPORTANT

I want to start by building a strong foundation for you. When it comes to conquering ED there are several aspects that are important. One of the most important is proper breathing.

The first step you can take to become a more sexually powerful person is learning to breathe properly. Breathing correctly is essential if you want to enhance your sexual performance. Correct breathing may not sound like a big deal to you right now, but when it comes to your sexual performance, it truly is a biggie.

Many of the exercises you are going to be learning in this book will require breath control. Doing these exercises will be much easier and <u>considerably more effective</u> if you learn to breathe properly.

The way you breathe affects you in many ways. It affects the way you move, stand, and how you perceive yourself. And how the world perceives you will mirror how you see yourself. Before the world can see you as being sexually powerful, you must see yourself as being sexually powerful. Only then will it radiate out into the world.

Types of Breathing

There are two types of breathing, chest breathing, and abdominal breathing. If you breathe using only your chest this will leave the lower part of your lungs blocked or immobilized. However, when you breathe using your abdomen the air that has been trapped at the bottom of the lungs with will be replaced with fresh clean air.

Here is an interesting fact you probably didn't realize... It takes approximately 3 chest breaths to get as much oxygen into the body as 1 abdominal breath. Unfortunately, most people are not in the habit of using their abdomen which allows them to breathe deeply. This is also the natural way to breathe.

The next time you get a chance, watch a newborn baby breathe. You will see their abdomen moving up and down. The truth is, you were born knowing how to properly breathe, but people tend to forget it as they get older. As a result, we must learn abdominal breathing all over again.

Correct breathing enhances the body's supply of energy that flows through it. This works in much the same way that diet enhances the body's store of essential nutrients.

Being able to control your breathing will open energy pathways (which you will learn more about a little later). It will improve your erection, and it will expand the feeling of your orgasm.

So, why does it work? Abdominal breathing sends energy down and through the urogenital diaphragm and that relaxes the pelvic floor. We will cover the pelvic floor and sexual energy a little later in the book.

Without deep breathing the lower abdomen tends to be tight. This tightness can lead to premature ejaculation, impotence, and sexual frustration.

As a bonus, proper breathing can help control stress. When someone is in a stressful situation, they tend to take short shallow gasps of air. This allows air to get stuck in their chest. Proper breathing allows oxygen to flow freely through the body which helps reduce stress. And we all know that stress can be a real killer for your sex drive.

The Anatomy of Breathing

This is not going to be a long-drawn-out anatomy lesson, just a quick overview so you can see how deep breathing works.

I'm not sure you ever thought about it, but the average person breathes between 20,000 and 23,000 times every day. (Just a random fact. in case you are at a cocktail party and need something to talk about.)

There are, however, several things that may cause a person to fall into "less-than-optimal" breathing patterns. These includes such things as:

- Stress
- Increased time sitting
- Poor posture

A less-than-optimal breathing pattern usually involves having a poor posture. This includes having the shoulders rounded and the head forward, and a slight hunch to the upper back.

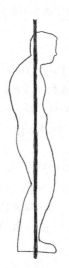

In your body there is a large respiratory muscle called the diaphragm. When you are in this posture, with your head forward, it is difficult for the diaphragm to fully engage. (This will also be covered in another chapter)

But air must get air into your lungs somehow. The way this is typically accomplished is by the muscles of the neck and shoulders pulling the rib cage up. This allows the rib cage and lungs to expand.

The problem is this pulling up lowers the air pressure in the chest so that air enters by suction. This suction leaves the lower part of the lungs empty.

Over time, this can lead to neck and upper back tension and pain as well as several other health-related issues, such as:

- Elevated blood pressure
- Increased heart rate
- Chronic stress
- Anxiety
- Poor posture
- Headaches
- Restricted range of motion of the upper back and shoulders

How you breathe will affect the overall feeling of the body. Your breathing will either empower you or it will deprive you of the power you need to look and feel confident.

Proper breathing should employ three areas of the lungs in a smooth and unbroken movement. Proper breathing begins in the abdomen and not in the chest. The bottom (of the lungs) is the first to fill with air, followed by the middle, and lastly the top of the lungs.

When your diaphragm is in its normal position, which is up, the lower part of your lungs is compressed. This compression prevents air from entering that part of your lungs. But when the diaphragm is pushed down the lower part of the lungs is allowed to expand, which allows it to fill with air.

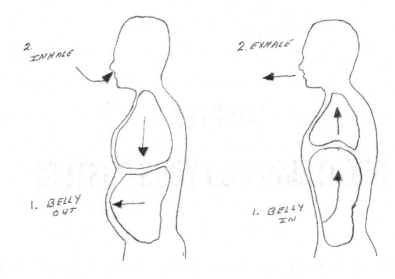

In this diagram you can see how the diaphragm goes down and the belly pushes out as the air enters the lungs. (This is exaggerated in the diagram. You don't have to push your belly out like this when you do abdominal breathing.) When you exhale the diaphragm moves up to its natural position and the air escapes out.

Incorporating this type of breathing into your daily routine can have a tremendous impact on both your overall well-being and your sexual life.

A little later, you are going to spend some time practicing deep abdominal breathing, but first I wanted to give you a little insight on the proper way to breathe.

In the next chapter, we are going to expand on your breathing as well as proper posture, which is essential for proper breathing.

Don't forget, everything you are doing here is going to have a tremendous effect on your sexual performance. You are not just killing time with these breathing lessons. What you are learning here is going to pay off more than you can imagine.

CHAPTER 2

BREATHING AND YOUR POSTURE

In this chapter we are going to talk about your sexual magnetism and something that will have a <u>profound</u> effect on it.

I'm talking about your posture and how your posture presents you to the world. You never get a second chance to make a first impression, so let's make that first impression the right one.

One of the first things a person notices about you is your posture. You can have great clothes and hair, but if your posture is poor, you are <u>not</u> going to make the best first impression.

For example, look at the difference between Superman and Clark Kent. They had very distinct postures. Clark had rounded shoulders and his head jutted forward. Because of this, he looked like a man who was lacking confidence. Let's face it, the girls were NOT rushing to get a date with Clark Kent.

But, when he changed into Superman, he threw his shoulders back which puffed out his chest. Immediately strength and confidence radiated from him. So, unless you are a superhero in disguise the Clark Kent persona is not one you want to project.

Paying attention to these two things, you're breathing and your posture, will allow you to project confidence, strength, and sexuality.

Poor posture effects your skeleton and it impacts the most important thing you do: your breathing.

Consider this: poor posture can affect your ability to breathe by up to 30%. Would you go to the gym every day and work out for an hour if you knew that 20 minutes of that hour was wasted and not doing anything for you? I realize this is only an example, but it is an accurate one.

Perhaps it doesn't seem possible to you that the position of your head, neck, shoulders, and back can influence your breathing. Consider this; Your head alone normally weighs between 10 and 12 pounds.

When your body isn't supporting it as well as it should, the rest of your physical functions are thrown out of whack!

Let me ask you a few questions.

Do you spend more than two hours a day in your car?

Do hours pass by as you hunch over your laptop?

Do you spend hours in the evening looking at social media on your cell phone?

If you said yes to even one of these questions, then your posture probably needs some work. The good news is that I'm going to give you the basics of fixing your posture.

Here is something you may have never heard of; it's called Forward Head Position (FHP). This comes from doing the things I just mentioned:

Texting with your cell phone

Driving for several hours

Surfing the web on your phone or tablet

Having your head constantly looking down at that angle, can position your ears roughly 4 ½ inches in front of your shoulders. They should be aligned directly above your shoulders.

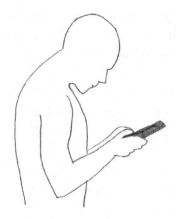

In the ideal posture your head is positioned with your ears over your shoulders. Your shoulders are aligned with your hips. Your hips are aligned with your knees. And your knees are aligned with your ankles.

According to Chiropractors, for every inch your head moves forward, 10 pounds in weight is added to your upper back and neck muscles. Adding the extra weight requires your muscles to work harder to support your head.

Your skeleton, shoulders, and neck muscles are not the only things affected by poor posture. In fact, poor posture blocks the action of the intercostal muscles (the muscles between your ribs) that <u>naturally</u> lift your ribs during inhalation. As a result, you squeeze your lungs and other organs into a cramped position which in turn limits the ability of your diaphragm to do its job.

Do you think about your posture, and then try to "get it right"? If so, you probably present a "stiff" pose that doesn't look natural. If you fall into this category, <u>let's work on fixing these it right now.</u>

Here is step one.

The first thing I want you to do is get a picture of yourself from the side. Do this from both a sitting and standing position. Don't change your posture in any way from what it usually is.

Now, look at the pictures.

Is the back of your head in line with your spine or is it leaning forward?

Is your back curved?

If so, let's make a few adjustments

First, I want you to gently push your chin back slightly, so your ears are directly over your shoulders.

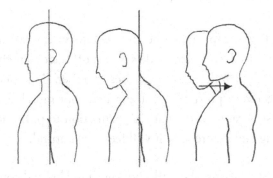

Now, take another picture. Did you Notice how much of a difference that one thing made? One simple adjustment can make a big difference in your appearance

Let's move to step 2

In step two we will be working with the shoulders. Go back to the pictures you took in step one and look at the position of your shoulders.

Next, I want you to move over to a wall and stand with your back against the wall. Your shoulder blades should be flat against the wall.

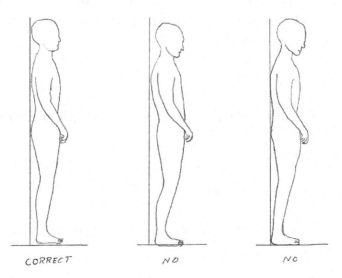

CORRECT   NO   NO

If they are not, you can make one simple adjustment, so they are. The most common mistake a person makes is to "puff" out your chest. Instead, I want you to slide your shoulder blades together. This one movement will help correct your posture and strengthen your muscles. This may be difficult at first because of the natural inclination to puff out your chest. Keep practicing and before long it will feel very natural.

While you are still against the wall, slide one hand behind your lower back so you can gauge how much space there is between the curve of your lower back and the wall. Ideally there should be just enough space to allow you to slide your hand through easily.

If there is too much space, tilting your hips forward will narrow it. If, however, it is too tight tilt your butt backward. This will create more curve at the back of your spine. This is not as easy to do as it sounds.

In fact, you may need someone to help you with this. I know because when I first started doing this, it made my lower back hurt. Then I found out that I was doing it incorrectly. With that in mind, I am going to try to explain how to do it correctly.

First, don't think of your hips as "thrusting" forward and backward. Instead, think of them as swiveling on a ball joint. When you tilt it, you are either pulling your pelvic bone up or pushing it down depending on which way you want the hip to tilt.

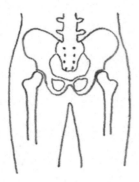

Tilting your pelvis will make a difference in the distance between your lower back and the wall. It will also make a difference in how you feel.

Next, while you are still standing against the wall see if your back and head are against the wall. If not, move them back so they are. If this alignment makes you feel as if you are leaning back, it is probably because you have been leaning forward for so long.

Having rounded shoulders also contracts and constricts your pectoral muscles. Again, this is usually due to prolonged driving, computers, and other devices we look at every day.

The best solution to this problem is deep tissue massage and stretching. One way to stretch is to lie down with a tennis ball under your back and move so the tennis ball rolls around under your back. Another way is to lie down with a rolled towel under your upper back.

Let's take a minute and talk about the complications of having poor posture. Poor posture can lead to weakness and instability. This can lead to the deterioration of spinal joints and eventually degenerative joint disease. Which is severe arthritis of the spine.

Proper posture and breathing can affect your sex life as well as your quality of life.

In the next chapter we will go through the process of abdominal breathing.

CHAPTER 3

ABDOMINAL BREATHING

I want to start this chapter with something I said before, one complete abdominal breath should employ 3 areas of your lungs in a smooth, unbroken movement that begins in the abdomen and not in the chest.

For this to happen you must use your diaphragm. Again, breathing without using the diaphragm immobilizes the lower part of your lungs, which in turn deprives your body of oxygen.

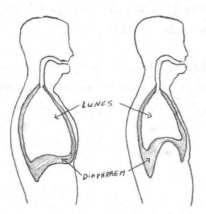

You can perform one simple test to tell if you are chest breathing or if you are using your diaphragm. Put one hand on your chest and the other on your stomach. Now, take a normal breath. If the hand on your chest moves before the hand on your stomach you are doing chest breathing.

You can perform proper abdominal breathing by relaxing your chest and breathing in deeply drawing air into your abdomen. You should feel your abdomen expanding in the front, back, and sides. This will allow your lungs to fill from the bottom first then up to the top.

Let's walk through the steps so you can learn how to properly perform abdominal breathing. Don't forget, proper breathing is the first step you must take to enhance your sexual performance.

This is important, so you want to get it right.

1) Slowly inhale air through your nose. Allow it flow into the lower lungs by letting the diaphragm expand and balloon downwards into your abdominal cavity.

As the diaphragm moves downward, your stomach should push out slightly. When you are first learning, you may want to gently push your stomach out. Doing this will help your body get used to the movement. Do not over-extend your stomach by pushing it out as far as you can. This can cause problems such as light-headedness.

Remember, this is the natural way to breathe and should require little effort on your part once you relearn the basics.

2) When the diaphragm is fully expanded the intercostal muscles (which are the muscles between the ribs) will naturally start to open the rib cage. This will allow the middle part of the lungs to fill with air.

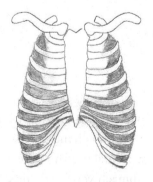

3) As you feel the rib cage reaching full capacity, gently lift your clavicles (collarbone). This will allow air to flow into the upper part of the lungs.

4) As you exhale things will happen in the exact opposite order. The collarbone will come down as air is released from the upper lungs.

5) The air from the chest will come out and finally, the air from the bottom of the lungs will escape as you gently pull your stomach in.

When you use abdominal breathing your body will automatically start to relaxed and be calm.

There are also other benefits of abdominal breathing such as:

- Reducing stress
- Activating the cranial and sacral pumps (we will get into both later)
- Keeping the spinal cord fluid moving and flowing in the joints and cranium
- Increasing your sexual energy

Without abdominal breathing, the lower abdomen tends to become tight and constricted. This tightness and constriction causes an imbalance in the sexual area. This imbalance can lead to low sexual energy which can cause:

Premature ejaculation

Wet dreams

Impotence and sexual frustration

Before I end this chapter, I want to talk about one more thing: It's called Reverse Breathing

Reverse breathing is just what it sounds like. It is doing the abdominal breathing in reverse. Instead of the stomach going out when you are breathing in, you pull the stomach in.

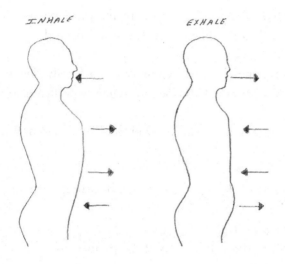

Now...A Word of Caution

Some martial arts practitioners feel reverse breathing is dangerous. They feel that the manipulation of breath should be reserved for hard-core qigong and advanced internal arts users.

They advise against attempting reverse breathing until you are <u>very</u> comfortable with abdominal breathing.

Another aspect we haven't touched on yet is where to place your attention. When working with your body's internal energy, where you place your attention (your focus) and your intent is very important. We will cover this in more detail later.

As another word of caution, if your attention and intent is not observed, or is incorrect, you could lose your energy instead of enhancing it. Even worse, you might tense your face, neck, and chest. You could also draw your diaphragm <u>upward</u> as you inhale, and that could lead to a variety of problems including chest pain, diarrhea, increased heart rate, and increased blood pressure.

As you can see, this is not something you should take lightly. AGAIN, DO NOT TRY THIS UNTIL YOU ARE VERY COMFORTABLE WITH ABDOMINAL BREATHING.

Here are the steps involved in reverse breathing.

1) Inhale slowly and pull the lower abdomen toward the spine. As you do this, you should feel a downward pressure between the back of your sexual organs and your anus (your perineum).

2) Pull up on your perineum and sexual organs while you simultaneously push down and lower your diaphragm.

3) Exhale and release your sexual organs and diaphragm allowing it to expand on all sides.

Using reverse breathing will help sync the life-force energy (Qi) in your body, thereby improving balance and stability.

If you decide you want to try reverse breathing, first get very comfortable with abdominal breathing.

Then find a comfortable place to sit with your spine in an upright position.

Keep the tip of your tongue in gentle contact with the roof of your mouth (behind the front teeth) and slightly tuck your chin so your ears are over your shoulders.

Close your eyes and place your hands in a triangle shape over your lower abdomen, with the tips of the thumbs touching, just over the navel.

As you inhale, pull the lowest portion of your abdomen (the part between the tips of your four fingers) gently inward towards your spine, away from your hands.

W. R. Mills

Exhale through your mouth and allow your abdomen to naturally expand outward back to its starting position.

The pressure should be extremely gentle.

Again, practice deep abdominal breathing first, and if you feel up to it, practice reverse breathing. These two types of breathing will have a tremendous impact on your sexual energy.

As with anything new, proceed slowly, mindfully, and practice in moderation.

CHAPTER 4

BREATHING AND NITRIC OXIDE

We have covered a lot of ground when it comes to breathing. But there are a couple more very important parts of your sexual enhancement I need to make sure you understand

First, I want to talk to you about Nitric Oxide. Not to be confused with Nitrous Oxide which is used to make race cars go faster or to ease your pain at the dentist's office. Nitric Oxide, on the other hand, will allow you to have and maintain a greater erection.

Nitric oxide is a naturally occurring gas, no not that kind of gas. This gas is secreted by cells which line the inner walls of blood vessels and help increase blood flow.

It is also a vasodilator meaning it relaxes the inner muscles of blood vessels, causing them to widen. You need Nitric oxide for the muscles in your penis to relax. This relaxation allows the chambers inside the penis to fill with blood so the penis can become erect.

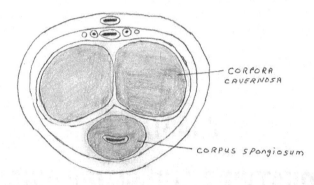

So, if you're ready to give your sex life and your erection a boost, let's look at you and Nitric Oxide.

The first question you are probably wondering is: If it is so important, can I increase my Nitric Oxide? The answer is yes. And I am going to tell you how you can do just that.

First, you start with a healthy lifestyle. Heart-healthy exercise releases nitric oxide. Lowering your cholesterol and your high blood pressure will also help. Decreasing your emotional stress will help. (We have already talked about how controlling your breathing can help with reducing your stress)

The second way to increase nitric oxide is with a healthy diet. Here are some great food sources for increasing nitric oxide:

- L-arginine is an amino acid, that's a protein building block, which is found in poultry, fish, red meats, and dairy products
- L-citrulline: is also an amino acid found in meat, nuts, legumes (a plant in the pea family), and watermelon
- The other source for increasing nitric oxide is dietary nitrates found in foods like beets, radishes, and dark leafy greens like spinach lettuce, and Kale.

Third, another great way to increase Nitric Oxide is breathing through your nose. Enzymes have been found in the nose and in the sinuses that produce Nitric Oxide.

According to an article in the American Journal of Respiratory and Critical Care Medicine, the main production of Nitric Oxide is in the sinuses with some also being produced in the nose. It was also found that humming increased the production of nitric oxide in the nasal cavity.

If you were to ask most people if they breathe through their mouth or their nose they will say through their nose, but generally, this is not true. If you observe those around you, you will see that a large percentage of people are mouth breathers.

Breathing through your nose is one of the most beneficial things you can do for the overall health of your body and your sex life.

Let me simplify why mouth breathing is bad.

Breathing should be very passive, and with little effort. We should not hear or notice someone breathing. Breathing heavily causes your blood vessels to constrict and that restricts the flow of blood up to your brain <u>by up to 50%.</u> This is one reason mouth breathers tire easily.

Also mouth breathing does not let our bodies take advantage of the sinuses production of Nitric Oxide.

We discussed earlier that most people breathe incorrectly. They either mouth breathe, or they chest breathe. Our bodies require a certain amount of oxygen. However, you are not getting enough for your brain, your heart, and other organs when you are breathing through your mouth. If you keep in mind the function of each of our organs, then it becomes quite simple.

You use your mouth to eat and talk and you use your nose to smell and breathe.

The more you breathe through your nose, the more Nitric Oxide you produce and the better your sex life.

The second thing I want to talk to you about is your breathing and your sex life. It's no secret that deep abdominal breathing, which can be considered a type of meditation, has its benefits.

Let's go over a few of the basics again.

> Better oxygen flow
> Helps you live free from anxiety
> Helps you relax
> Helps improves sleep
> Puts you in a better mood
> Improves your state of mind
> Moves fresh oxygenated blood into the heart
> Enhances your sexual pleasure

If you follow the practice of abdominal breathing, you will see how controlling your breathing will make you feel better, increase you sex drive, have better orgasms, increase your endurance, and connect more deeply with your partner.

When I was younger, I can remember becoming sexually aroused almost instantly, but that isn't necessarily true as you get older. Sometimes you get wrapped up in your own head…

Will my erection be hard enough?

Will it last long enough to satisfy my partner?

Clearing your mind is necessary for focusing on giving and receiving sexual pleasure. Taking controlled deep breaths will clear your mind and put you in a more relaxed mood.

There are reasons why Yoga, Qigong, and meditations focus so heavily on breathing. Controlled breathing calms the body. As you calm down, you become more aware. You are more aware of your body, more aware of what's occurring around you, and how something makes you feel.

Focused breathing helps take you away from worrying and helps center you. In fact, rhythmic breathing can be so incredibly powerful that you can technically achieve an orgasm while running, meditating, or even swimming.

But it doesn't stop there. Holding your breath reduces the amount of oxygen arriving at the muscles your body is using; it makes you tired faster. As a result, your energy levels can dip, your erection can soften, your arousal can lessen, and the sex will end faster.

On the other hand, controlling your breathing will help prolong sex, keep you harder longer, delay your orgasms, and make your climax more intense when it arrives.

Oxygen also gets you high. Deep breathing during sex elevates the sensation of euphoria. Therefore, the more you breathe, the better you feel, and the better you feel, the better the sex.

Deep breathing into the belly increases blood flow around your entire body. Your touch receptors will activate, resulting in the enhancement of sexual pleasure.

You can control your breathing and focus on it. You <u>can</u> modify your breathing to change what's happening in your body. With your breathing, you can control stress and fear, <u>and</u> you can also control your sexual arousal which lets you last longer during sex.

Now, let's go over the breathing techniques you can use to Increase your bedroom stamina.

In this exercise, I want you to stop what you are doing and simply put all your attention on your breathing.

Focus on your inhalations and your exhalations

Inhale through your nose. Let the fresh oxygen fill your abdomen and up to your chest and to the very top of your lungs.

Exhale and let the air flow out of your body.

You will notice how focusing on your breathing automatically makes you breathe more slowly and deeply. Just after a few breaths you already feel more relaxed. The more relaxed you are, the more in control you are of what's happening in your body.

Take a few more deep breaths. focus only on your breathing.

Visualize the air first filling your belly, then rising to your rib cage, then to your heart and then to your throat; be aware of those 4 points as you inhale.

When you exhale, just let go of all the air and relax. Don't force the air out of your lungs but just let it go. Make the sound "haaaaaaa" as you release the air. We will go over why this is important in a later chapter.

Now that you know that breathing is one of the keys to controlling your climax, you can incorporate it into your sexual practice. This can be done when you masturbate, or during intercourse. Focus on your body and the sensations you are feeling.

Also, be aware of your arousal and where you are on a scale of 1 to 10; you should be able to focus on this and on your breathing at the same time.

Whenever you feel your arousal going up faster than you would like, focus on your breathing, and start doing deep breathing as I just described. This alone will bring your arousal back down and give you more control.

There's nothing wrong with focusing on your breathing or using deep breathing while making love. It will help you last longer.

I have also seen this happen. If you only focus on your breathing and forget about the sex you are having, it can bring your arousal down too much and you can lose your erection. So, take a couple of seconds to focus on your breathing to draw you away from the impending climax, then back to the sex.

To summarize, when you feel your arousal going up, focus on your breathing, slow down your breathing, and breathe fully starting by filling the belly. This will bring your arousal back down and keep you in control.

Here is something to keep in mind.

If you're looking for a magic pill that solves all your sexual problems with no effort on your part, I'm sorry to tell you that such a thing doesn't exist.

Like anything of value in life, learning how to extend your lovemaking sessions requires some work. But controlling your breathing really is the closest thing there is to a magic pill.

CHAPTER 5

ENERGY BREATHING

In this chapter we are going to look at energy breathing.

Energy breathing is different from abdominal breathing. It is designed to create efficient circulation and strengthen the energy in the lower abdominal area.

This "energy breath" is performed by rapidly expelling the air out of the lungs. It is easy to do physically but it may require some practice to do it mentally. I only say that because for this practice to work you will need to do some visualization.

We will go into visualization in more detail in the next chapter, but I want you to start getting some practice with it now.

I want you to practice visualizing this exercise before you try to do it.

First, I want you to visualize, or imagine, a small fire directly behind your navel. I want you to close your eyes for a few seconds and "see" a flame start to form in your abdomen.

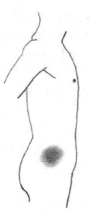

The only thing this flame needs to turn into a brilliant fire is air. I want you to see yourself blowing air into this flame to make it spring into a giant fire. If you were a blacksmith, you would use a bellow to blow air into fire to make it hotter and increase the flame. As you breathe air into the flame, I want you to make the same sound you would hear if you were in a blacksmiths shop. If you are not sure what that sounds like, use the sound you would make if you were starting a fire and were blowing on it to make it larger.

Making this sound may seem silly, but it is actually very important. It is easier to visualize it happening if you make the sound.

Continue to visualize the fire. Then watch yourself forcefully expelling all the air from your lungs using a strong contraction of the abdominal wall.

Immediately after you expel the air, see your lungs filling naturally with air until they are about half full.

When the lungs are half full, see yourself immediately contracting your abdomen wall again and forcefully expelling another gust of air. Every time you expel the air see the flame getting larger.

Every time you visualize yourself expelling the air, physically make the sound of blowing on the flame.

This exercise will strengthen and energize your lower abdominal area where your sexual energy lies. Continue doing this part until you can vividly see the flame in your mind growing into a large flame.

Now that you have visualized it, let's try it and see if you can get the internal energy flame blazing.

Close your eyes and try to visualize a small fire directly behind your naval. Concentrate on the area just behind your naval. In your mind, see the small fire starting to glow.

When you can see the fire in your mind's eye, take a breath and see yourself blowing directly on the fire. Forcefully exhale the air by contracting your abdomen while you are making the blowing sound.

Let your lungs fill with air until they are about half full. Then immediately contract the abdominal wall and forcefully blow the air out of your lungs while making the blowing sound.

Let your lungs fill halfway with air again and then forcefully blow the air out again while making the blowing sound.

Doing 2 breaths should be enough for your first try. Don't overdo this exercise. Go slowly with this and don't try to rush it. Slowly build up until you can do 20 – 30 of them.

Do NOT Rush This.

It will take time and practice to work your way up to the 20 -30 energy breaths. Besides that, it will take some practice for you to be able to visualize the flame.

Instead of rushing to do the exercises, spend some time practicing trying to visualize the small fire behind your naval.

Work on completing this assignment and when you have, move on to the next chapter.

PART 2

MINDSET AND VISUALIZATION

CHAPTER 6

MINDSET

In this chapter we are going to address something that has the potential to change your life forever.

When you started this book, one of the first things I said to you was that on some level, I believe everyone wants to change their reality.

This could be the way we:

Think

React to different situations

Cope with stress

Interact and communicate with others

Manage our fears

The fact that our sex life isn't what it used to be

I said "we" because no one is immune to this. I fall right into the same category. So, let me ask you, are there things you would like to change about yourself? Do you want to become a better version of yourself?

Deep down, I believe everyone wants to learn, grow, and evolve. That's why people spend $10 Billion a year on personal development products and programs.

If a new reality is what you desire, what are the quickest ways to create this new reality?

The first step is: <u>Change comes from Believing</u>.
The second step is: <u>Change Comes from Doing</u>.

I want you to discover the powerful impact "mindset" has on your life. There are 2 types of mindsets, or attitudes if you prefer.

One of the hardest things to understand is the fact that it is not <u>just</u> your abilities and talents that bring you success. Instead, it is whether you approach things with a fixed or a growth mindset. The success is am talking about might be in your business life, your personal life, or in your sexual life.

People who have a <u>growth</u> mindset believe that basic qualities, like your intelligence, can be strengthened just like muscles can be strengthened. Growth-minded people seek out opportunities for improvement. They also take on challenges to better their circumstances.

On the other hand, people with a fixed mindset believe they are not going to get any better than they are right now. Therefore, they have little incentive to work hard. Why bother to put in a little effort to build something if you are convinced you can't do it, and you believe there is nothing you can do to change it?

You, more than likely, do not have a straight fixed-mindset or growth-mindset, you are a little of both. You will probably find there are some things you do with a growth mindset (where you are trying to improve yourself) and other things you do with a fixed mindset (believing you can't change what you are).

This realization alone can have an impact on the way you approach everything in life. This may seem like just a lot of talk but keep reading and let me back it up.

Let me tell you a little about myself.

I grew up in a small town. My dad worked two jobs and was very seldom at home. I was the youngest of four and the only boy. It was a rough neighborhood, and I was about the only boy in the neighborhood who had not been arrested.

We were poor but being young I didn't realize it. I thought everyone was just like us. After I started school, I found out that things were not the way I assumed they were.

So at 12 I got my first job delivering newspapers after school. I worked 6 days a week every week. Work was never called off because of rain, snow, or ice. If you had a paper route, you delivered papers.

In the winter I often couldn't feel my feet because all I had was rain boots, not warm winter boots, and in the winter, I didn't get finished with my route until after dark.

Besides delivering the newspaper, I also had to collect the payments due from my customers so I could pay the bill at the newspaper office. If everyone paid their bill, and that rarely happened, I made 8 dollars a week.

When I turned 16, I got a job working for that same newspaper handing out the papers to the kids who delivered them. I also cleaned the office after they closed. I did that 6 days a week until I turned 18 and was old enough to get a job at a metal recycling plant in our town.

At 19 I got married and had 2 children. It sounded like a lot of fun at the time. Until I dropped out of the trade school I was enrolled in. It turns out that having a wife and kids was expensive.

My family and I went back to our hometown, and I got a job at the paper mill. A few years later, my dad died, and I decided to continue the business he started, so I quit my job at the factory. I was 26.

I didn't know anything about running a business and it wasn't long before I lost our house and what little savings we had. I decided that was never going to happen again, boy was I wrong. I repeated this cycle two more times.

Just wanting something wasn't enough, I had to learn how to run a business. I spent my spare time studying and learning. The next business I started lasted over 30 years and it was quite lucrative.

I believed I could do it, I wanted it, but it wasn't until I made myself study and learn how to run a business that it succeeded.

You purchased this book with the plan that you could change something. You wanted the change and believing you could make the change was the first step.

What you will learn in this book will teach you how to complete this process. This is true for your sex life and every other part of your life.

Nothing comes for free!

You will have to work for it, perform the exercises and follow the advice you are given. Stick with it and you <u>will</u> get the results you want.

That is what mindset is all about.

Here are some potential life-altering ideas that will help you on your journey

1) If you currently have a fixed mindset and believe you are stuck with your situation, there is good news. It's not a permanent thing. You can change it and develop a growth mindset.

Not only is mindset an important part of life in general, it is an important part of your sex life. and you can change your mindset.

2) Focus on learning instead of achievement. As you go through this book, focus on your growth instead of focusing on your achievements alone. The more you embrace the ideas presented to you and implement them into your life, the faster the achievements will come.

I want you to learn about your brain and all the ways it can help you grow and overcome obstacles (such as getting rid of the effects of ED). Every time you do something that is new, and stick to it, your brain forms stronger and stronger connections, and over time your abilities will grow.

3) Learn to love the process of growing. Celebrate every progress you make along the way, no matter how small. There will be challenges because you will be doing, and learning, things you have not done before.

4) Work on your physical and creative abilities. Just because some people seem naturally good at something, does not mean others can't do it. In fact, with the proper training, others can do it even better.

Let me give you an example. Listen to the story of Wilma Rudolph. Wilma was not a physical wonder as a young child. She was a premature baby; she was the twentieth of twenty-two children and she was constantly sick.

When she was 4 she almost died. She had double pneumonia, scarlet fever, and polio. She did survive but her left leg was mostly paralyzed. Doctors gave her little hope of ever using it again.

For eight years, she worked with physical therapy. She was 12 years old when she was finally able to remove her leg brace. Her story could end there, and it would be quite a story, but it doesn't.

You see, Wilma was hailed as the fastest woman on earth after she won three gold medals for sprints and relays in the 1960 Rome Olympics.

5) Understand that the journey is the ultimate reward not overcoming your ED. I realize you are so concerned with overcoming your ED that nothing else seems important. I don't want you to get the impression that the desired outcome (conquering your ED) isn't going to happen. That is not what I mean. I mean you will grow considerably getting to the outcome.

You are going to grow in so many ways as you go through this book. Your sexual abilities are going to skyrocket. The pleasure you are going to give your partner is going to go through the roof. But you need to have the right mindset.

You must believe you can do it, but then you must go further. You must do the exercises. You must listen to what you are being told. It will be easy to skip the exercises and the practices.

I get that you are busy. But then you will wonder why everything I promised is not happening. Look, I can't make you do the exercise, I can't make you practice, and I can't make you believe.

But I can do this.

I will tell you the truth. And everything I am going to teach you has worked for thousands of years.

Work through this book and master each section and it will work for you.

In the next chapter, we are going to go further into the power you hold in your mind.

CHAPTER 7

VISUALIZATION

In this chapter, we are going to discuss visualization which works along with mindset. These two things, mindset and visualization, are going to work together throughout this entire book.

Visualization is a technique that uses your imagination, mental images, and the power of thought to make your dreams and goals come true. Used in the right way, visualization can improve every aspect of your life and your love life.

Visualization is <u>power</u> and it can alter your environment and circumstances. Visualization can also <u>cause</u> events to happen.

By visualizing a certain event, situation, or object, you attract it into your life. For some people, this might sound like magic, but there is no magic involved, only the natural process of the power of thoughts and natural mental laws.

You may be thinking this is just a bunch of new-age, hippy-dippy stuff, but I can assure you it isn't. In fact, we are going to look at the actual science behind it in a few minutes.

Almost everyone, even if you are not a religious or a spiritual person, more than likely believes in a power higher than themselves. You may call this power God, or the Universal Mind, or a higher consciousness. In fact, this power has many names, depending on where you are located and your personal beliefs.

So, I present this thought to you... If everything that exists came from this power (or energy) this power must be <u>in</u> everything that exists. Therefore, everything that exists must be a part of this power.

That includes you. You are part of this power. You have this power running through you. All you must do is tap into it.

The energy that is alive and circulating inside of you is the same energy that created everything that exists. Think about this; This allows <u>you</u> to participate in the creation process. This is one of the reasons that thoughts materialize.

Give this a moment to sink in... Your thoughts can come true!

That doesn't mean that every thought you have is going to come true. But the thoughts that are focused, well-defined, and often repeated can come true.

Your thoughts are energy. This energy will be even stronger if the thought is empowered with emotional energy. Your thoughts can change the balance of the energy around you. That in turn, brings changes to the environment around you.

New research coming out of Oxford and Cambridge, suggests that your ability to vividly imagine details about a bright future dramatically increases your energy. When your mind's eye can picture exactly what that bright future looks like, it can orient itself in the direction of what you envision. The more vividly you can picture something, the more attainable it feels.

As an example, research has found that if you visualize making a shot in basketball the likelihood of you making it goes slightly up. If you <u>visualize</u> waking up at 5 A.M. to practice, <u>visualize</u> working on your form, and <u>visualize</u> the feel of the ball in your hands right before it leaves for the basket, the likelihood of you making the shot rises even more. The more vivid your visualization, the more real it feels. And research shows the more real it feels, the more likely it will be to impact your behavior.

Once you recognize this, you can begin to move to a world that gives you power!

There is a strong scientific basis for how and why visualization works. It is a well-known fact that we stimulate the same regions of the brain when we visualize an action as we do when we perform that same action.

For example, when you visualize lifting your foot, it stimulates the same part of the brain that is activated when you lift your foot. This has been demonstrated extensively in scientific literature.

There are also reports of how visualization increases brain activation in someone who has had a stroke. These reports were based on a person who had a stroke due to a blood clot in a brain artery. When this happens, blood cannot reach the tissue that the artery once fed and that tissue dies.

This "tissue death" then spreads to the surrounding area that no longer receives the blood. The report goes on to state that if the person with this stroke <u>imagines</u> moving the affected arm or leg, blood flow to the affected area of the brain increases, and the surrounding brain tissue is saved. Imagining moving a limb increases brain blood flow enough to diminish the amount of tissue death.

This is a very clear indicator of the power of visualization.

Athletes have known about this power for a long time. Studies show that when athletes first imagine obtaining their goal, whether it is shooting a basketball or running a race, in as much detail as possible, they are then able to execute it more efficiently after practicing visualizing it.

To cite a few of the many studies:

One study showed that youth soccer players increased their confidence in playing when they visualized their moves.

Visualization has also been shown to improve high jumpers clearing the bar.

Brain chemistry research has proven if you tell your brain your plan in words, it gets bored part-way through and wants to go to sleep. But if it sees it as a picture it will respond with much deeper interest and attention. As studies show, the images will get into your subconscious and help you to manifest them. Thereby you can convert your dreams to reality.

Let's look at your brain and visualization

The brain is constantly growing and expanding. Every time you learn something new, such as speaking a foreign language or learning how to change a tire on your car, you make an imprint in your brain, i.e., you make a memory. The more often you repeat or practice the task, the stronger the imprint becomes, and the easier it is to recall.

What the brain <u>can't</u> do is distinguish whether you are <u>physically experiencing something or simply imagining it</u>.

According to the International Coaching Academy's <u>neuroscience and visualization research paper</u>, "if you exercise an idea over and over in your mind, your brain will begin to respond as though the idea was a real object in the world." It is unfortunate the politicians also learned this… tell the people something long enough and they will believe it is real.

A study was done looking at brain patterns in weightlifters. It showed that the patterns activated when a weightlifter lifted hundreds of pounds were also activated when they only imagined lifting it.

Many athletes employ this technique, including Tiger Woods who has been using it since his pre-teen years.

Seasoned athletes use vivid, highly detailed visualizations and run-throughs of their entire performance. When they are doing their mental rehearsal, and they combine their knowledge of the sport with mental rehearsal for the best outcome.

World Champion Golfer, Jack Nicklaus has said: "I never hit a shot, not even in practice, without having a very sharp in-focus picture of it in my head."

Even heavyweight boxing champion Muhammad Ali used different mental practices to enhance his performance in the ring. He used visualization, mental rehearsal, self-confirmation, and perhaps the most powerful epigram of personal worth ever uttered: "I am the greatest.'"

I personally used this on every installation job I have done with my last business. I mentally did the entire job before I ever arrived on the job site. I had fewer problems and the jobs always went smoother.

In my personal life, after my wife died, I met the most beautiful woman, and I knew she was the one I was supposed to be with for the rest of my life. Every second of my spare time, I imagined us together living a wonderful life. It didn't happen overnight, but later she said yes and the "I do's" came shortly after that. It works for me, and thousands of successful people and it will work for you too.

Do not overlook the power of visualization. You have the power to change everything about you and your life right at your fingertips.

In the next chapter, you will start working with the process of visualization.

CHAPTER 8

USING VISUALIZATION

In the previous chapter we discussed what visualization is and why it works. In this chapter you are going to practice using it.

Here are the steps:

1) You must use a mental picture. Using words to describe the image won't work.

2) The image must be in as much detail as possible. Focus on the overall image and every small detail.

3) This must be something that has a strong emotional attachment to it. This will charge it with energy.

4) Play the scene out in your mind exactly as you want it to go.

5) As the scene plays out attach a strong <u>happy</u> emotion to it. This will help it cement into your subconscious mind.

6) The scene must "feel real" to you. You must "live" that scene in your mind. If you touch something or get touched, you must be able to feel that touch on your skin. If there is a smell, you must experience the

smell. If the sun is shining, feel the warm rays on your skin. If you are in bed, feel the texture of the sheets as your body touches it.

7) As your scene moves forward, feel the anticipation rising inside of you. Live every part of the scene all the way to the end. Experience every feeling just as you would if you were performing the action in real life. By doing this, you are training your mind and your body to work together.

Doing this one time, however, will not be enough for it to happen. Keep living this scene in your mind. The more you do it, the more your brain will believe it is happening. Like I said earlier, I did this for a few years, but it was so important to me that I continued doing it. And it came to pass!

Those are the steps, now you need to find something you are very passionate about, close your eyes and sit in a quiet place where you won't be disturbed. (Turn your phone off and relax).

Review the above steps if needed. Let the scene play out in your mind exactly as you want it to happen. You must feel every action just as if it was really happening.

Right now, you are probably most concerned with getting or keeping an erection. So, allow that scene to play out just as you want it to go. Make the scene as detailed as possible and feel it happening. Feel the touches on your skin, your lips, or all over your body. When the scene feels real, you will probably start to feel the arousal happening.

Keep practicing this until the scene feels real to you. Then continue doing this until it happens. After you have mastered how to visualize, proceed to the next chapter.

In recap:

In part 2 we talked about having the correct mindset and how to achieve it. If your mind is not set on growing, you will be stuck in the same rut you have lived in until <u>you</u> decide to change it.

First, you must believe it is possible to change (and it is).

Second, you need to take some action. The people who change, first believe they can change. That motivates them to act. You acted by purchasing this book and in the next section, you will continue to take more actions.

Next, we discussed the power of visualization. This is where the true magic happens. Your brain <u>cannot</u> tell the difference between doing something and imagining you are doing it. The only requirement is that it needs to feel real in your imagination for your brain to believe it.

Throughout this book, you will be asked to use visualization to help you achieve some of the objectives. If you start practicing it daily in every aspect of your life, changes in your life will come faster and easier.

Don't save visualization for the big things, start using it with every small thing you do. Go over every detail in your mind before you do it.

In the next section, we will start what I call Penis Enhancement Qigong. You will be learning how different parts of your body are tied together and how they work together to enhance your sexual life.

Once you have mastered this section, move on to the next part of the book. Don't make the mistake of just reading each chapter and then move along to the next one.

Practice and learn what is in each chapter before you move on to the next one.

PART 3

SECRET OF THE ORGANS

CHAPTER 9

MERIDIAN TRACING

I find it easier to connect with the exercises and maintain the repetition of the exercises if I understand how each organ connects with my body, my sexual center, and why I am doing something. Simply telling me to do something isn't good enough. I need to understand why I need to do it. So, before we start working with the organs, let's go over a few things.

The first written record we have of working with the energy in the body is approximately 2,000 years old and was written by the Chinese. They understood this very important principle: Everything that exists, when broken down, consists of energy and vibration. They also understood this energy is always in motion.

Energy continually circulates through your body. If it moves unhampered, you will remain healthy, both physically and sexually. But if the energy gets congested or blocked, your physical body, as well as your sexual prowess, is affected.

This internal energy moves along lines in the body called Meridians. These run from the top of your head to the bottom of your feet.

The meridians are a network of invisible pathways connecting to each other, each organ, every atom, cell, bone, muscle, tendon, and every part of your skin. Everything in your body is connected, nothing about your body is separate.

Not only is the physical body connected, your mind, emotions, and spirit are also connected.

There are 12 major meridians in the body, and they run on each side of the body. The left side and the right side, mirror each other. Each meridian also corresponds to an organ in the body. Each organ is dependent on the other organs that are along the meridian as well as the entire meridian network.

Energy flowing through the meridians is not the only function of the meridian. The meridians also transmit signals of information to the organs. This information is vital to keeping your body functioning properly. These signals are also essential for regulating your emotions. These energy pathways also help coordinate the work of the organs and help keep your body balanced by regulating its functions.

In later lessons, we will discuss this energy and its movement in our bodies in greater detail. For now, you need to realize there is an energy moving inside your body and it doesn't always move the way it should.

There are some things you can do to keep this energy moving correctly and you will start working with this in the next chapter.

The Chinese also believe our sexual prowess comes from five main organs:

The lungs

The heart

The liver

The kidneys

The spleen

Your goal will be to keep these organs in balance by keeping the energy flowing freely in your body. When the energy is flowing unobstructed these organs work in harmony. As a result, your body, mind, and spirit will be in balance. When "you" are in balance, your sexual energy will also be in balance.

With that being said, let's look at each of the five major organs and the associated meridians. We are not going to go into the acupuncture points, in this book, but I have included them in some of the images so you can see where they are located.

The Lungs:

The lungs are responsible for breathing and energy intake. A malfunctioning lung meridian results in more than just breathing problems. If the energy is not moving correctly through this meridian, you are susceptible to inflammation and infections. Your body also becomes open to skin diseases.

The Heart:

Obviously, the heart is essential to your health. It circulates blood to all the other organs in the body. If energy is not flowing correctly through this meridian, the results can be chest pains, irritability, and sleeplessness. This can also bring about mental and emotional disorders.

The Spleen:

The spleen ensures that the body gets enough nutrients, as well as regulating blood flow. A malfunctioning spleen meridian will result in digestive issues, weak muscles, fatigue, and brain fog.

The Liver:

The liver stores energy and controls how it flows through your body. A flaw in this meridian will cause your ligaments to become tense. It may also cause disorders like dry skin, vertigo, stiff joints, and headaches.

The Kidneys:

The kidneys provide your sexual energy. They also control how the reproductive system develops. This meridian is also responsible for bone marrow and blood flow. It also controls your willpower. If the energy flowing through this meridian is hampered, the result show up as genital disorders.

The Sex Meridian:

There is another meridian called the Sex Meridian (Pericardium) that envelops the heart. This meridian protects your heart both physically and emotionally. It lubricates the heart and draws any excess energy away from it. It also helps govern your circulation and hormones such as testosterone and estrogen. It also helps you connect love with sex.

The health of these organs and meridians directly affects your sexual energy. Your sexual energy is the essence of these organs. One example of this is that your body draws the finest energy from these organs to produce sperm.

If one or more of these organs is out of balance it has a direct effect on your sexual energy.

When it comes to meridians, there are two tools that are very helpful to re-establish balance in the meridians:

The meridian flush and meridian tracing.

Both methods involve following the outline of the meridian. You can follow the outline using one finger or you can use two or more fingers or your entire palm.

If you follow the meridian in the normal direction it flows, you will be tracing the meridian and strengthening it. Following it in the reverse direction will flush the meridian and will calm and sedate it.

Most people would think you should make the meridian stronger, but you will not always try to strengthen it. There are times when you will need to calm the meridian. What you are trying to achieve is balance.

Generally, if there is pain or inflammation along the meridian, or the organ it is associated with, this usually calls for calming or sedating the meridian. If there is coldness or weakness in the meridian or its associated organ, this calls for stimulation.

Here is the Meridian Tracing Technique:

Start the tracing by pausing your finger(s) or hand at the starting point of the meridian (Acupoint # 1). Then follow the meridian in an even and continuous motion. Your fingers or hand should be very close to your body. They can touch the skin, but it is not necessary.

You are working with energy, and energy can be manipulated by the energy coming from your fingers. It can also be manipulated by the energy coming from your mind when you visualize. There will be parts of the meridian where it goes internal, and you simply cannot touch it. When this happens, visualize the pathway, and then continue the tracing where it surfaces and you can reach the pathway.

When you need to repeat the tracing, such as after you perform a flushing, always move your hands back to the starting point.

You can trace the meridians every day or several times a day if you wish or simply do it weekly for maintenance. If you have meridians that need improvement, you may want to perform the tracing more frequently than once a week.

The Meridian Flush:

The meridian flush is basically a strong stimulation of a meridian. This will keep the flow open, calm the meridian, and prevent blockages.

If there is an unbalanced energy pattern of one organ, it is easily transmitted to other body parts that are on the pathway of the meridian. Therefore, it is important to keep the energy flowing and balanced by preventing blockages.

To flush a meridian, you trace it backwards once and then trace it forward 3 times.

There is one exception to the meridian flush rule. NEVER trace the heart meridian backward.

In the next Chapter, we'll start working on getting these organs in balance.

CHAPTER 10

KIDNEY MASSAGE

In this chapter we are going to work on your kidney energy system.

The kidneys are two bean-shaped organs, about the size of a fist, and are tucked slightly under the last rib, on each side of the spine. They are known as the Root-of-Life because the original prenatal energy which forms the basis of life is stored in the kidney energy system.

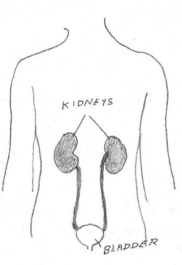

The kidneys are the body's most important reservoir of essential energy. The kidneys store reserve energy that is inherited from your parents, called "pre-natal Qi" (pronounced Chee). If another organ is low on energy, the kidneys will send it an extra energy boost from this reserve.

The kidneys also control sexual and reproductive functions and provide the body's main source of sexual vitality. Stimulating and energizing the kidneys is vital to having healthy sexual energy. I am going to show you two ways to stimulate and energize your kidneys.

One way to increase your kidney energy is by massage.

The kidneys are massaged from the back and this area of your back may be sensitive. I recommend that you use a good hand lotion for a few days to soften your hands before you perform these exercises.

First place the palms of both hands over the kidneys. Place one over each kidney on the lower back directly above the last rib. Begin to massage the kidney area.

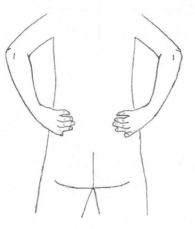

The idea is to generate heat for the kidneys. Continue massaging until you can feel the heat penetrating into your kidneys. Rub vigorously on the lower back, over the kidneys, and down to the sacrum, (your tailbone.) Rubbing vigorously does not mean rub hard. You are not trying to hurt yourself, just generate heat.

You will feel the entire area becoming energized. After you feel the heat and the area becoming energized, rest the palms of your hands directly over the kidneys and project energy from your hands into your kidneys and down to your tailbone.

Use your visualization method for projecting the energy into the kidneys. The energy you are projecting will come out of the palms of your hands as you project it. The more you work with your visualization, the easier it will be for you to project this energy.

Another good way to stimulate the kidneys is by gently tapping, or "knocking," the lower back area with a loose fist.

First locate the kidneys on the lower back like you did in the first method. Then make a loose fist and hit the kidneys using the flat part of the back of your fist, the part between the wrist and the knuckles. Don't use your knuckles. And you don't need to hit very hard. This should not feel uncomfortable. You are not trying to hurt yourself, only stimulate the kidneys.

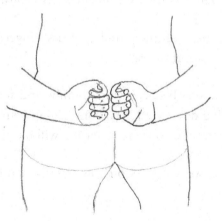

Alternate between hands, first knock with one fist on one kidney, and then with the other on the other kidney. Continue knocking all the way down to the tailbone. This should only take about 8 or 9 times and you will feel the vibration in the entire lower back area. After this, rub your palms together to warm them, then rub the palms up and down over the kidneys until they feel warm.

Next, you need to massage your ears. Yes, your ears. The ears are an extension of the kidney energy. By massaging the ears, you will stimulate even more energy into the kidneys.

When couples kiss and then nibble on their partner's ears, it is because the ears have more than 120 pressure points and stimulating them will directly activate their sexual energies.

In general, an ear massage will help your whole body. It will help every organ system, all the joints, <u>all</u> your body parts, and it will help keep your hearing healthy.

First if you are wearing earrings, take them off. Then using the two middle fingers, gently rub around and inside the entire ear several times.

Then place the palms of your hands over your ears and gently massage the ear using just enough pressure to stimulate energy in the entire ear.

Now place the ear between the thumb and first finger and rub the front of the ear and the back of the ear.

Next take each earlobe between your thumbs and forefingers and rub gently while pulling downward. Make massaging your ears part of your daily exercise routine and your sexual energy will increase.

In the next chapter we will work on how to trace and flush your kidney meridian.

CHAPTER 11

THE KIDNEY MERIDIAN

In this chapter, we are going to work with your Kidney Meridian.

This meridian is complex, so I am going to give you a simple version.

Don't forget, each meridian has two paths that mirror each other. One on the right side of the body and one on the left side of the body.

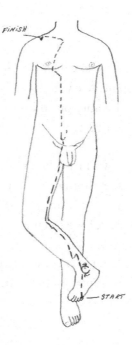

The Kidney Meridian begins under and on the inside of the little toe. From here it crosses the middle of the sole of your foot (at the arch). It then circles behind the inside of your ankle. From here it rises along the inner side of the leg up the calf and the inner thigh.

When it reaches the groin, it moves to the perineum, the point midway between your scrotum and your anus. From here it goes to the base of the spine, where it splits.

Part of it joins the Governing (also called the Governor channel) channel where it continues up the spine. We will discuss the governing channel in a later chapter. Right now, I want you to know that it is one of the two major energy channels in your body.

The other part of it connects with the kidney where it splits again. Part of it stays internal where it passes through several major organs such as the liver, the diaphragm, the lungs, the heart, the pericardium, and the throat before it terminates at the root of the tongue.

The other part comes out of the kidneys to the pubic bone. From here it comes over the abdomen and runs upward to the upper part of the chest ending at the collarbone.

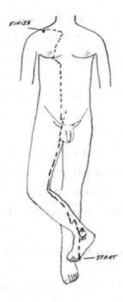

I stated in the last chapter that the kidneys store a reserve of energy that is used to supply a boost of energy if another organ is running low. Since this affects every organ in the body, it is <u>very important</u> to keep the energy in the kidney meridian balanced. You can trace the meridian to help balance the energy flowing in it.

Start with positioning your finger(s) along the inside and beneath the little toe and trace to the middle of the underside of the foot right in the middle of the ball of your foot.

From here, draw your fingers up behind your ankle bone (on the inside of the leg) and make a clockwise circle.

Move your palms up the inside middle of your leg all the way up to your groin. Using your fingers, trace the path until you touch your perineum. Again, that is the point half-way between your scrotum and your anus.

Mentally trace the pathway from your perineum to the tip of your tailbone and then straight forward to your pubic bone.

From here, continue to trace each meridian up the abdomen all the way to your chest and end at the collarbone. You can also use visualization to trace the branch from your tailbone up your spine to your neck and then use your fingers to trace it from your neck to the top of your head.

To flush the meridian, trace the meridian in the reverse order.

Start at your collarbone and follow the path down your chest all the way to your pubic bone. Mentally trace it back to your tailbone and then to your perineum.

Using your fingers, continue to follow the path to your groin.

Switch from your fingers to the palms of your hands and continue down the inside of your legs to your ankle.

At your ankle, switch to your fingers and make the counter-clockwise circle. Follow the path to the ball of your foot and then to the inside of your little toe.

To finish, trace the meridian forward three times.

You can do each leg separately or at the same time.

The massages you will be doing for the other organs will also indirectly massage the areas the kidney meridian passes through.

A final thought: kidneys are nourished through your Spleen/Stomach, meaning you must have a good diet and lifestyle to keep it healthy.

With that in mind, you should know that some foods are healthier for the kidneys and there are also some foods you should avoid. However, some of the foods that promote healthy kidneys may not be suitable for people with kidney disease. Always check with your doctor before you start a new diet or exercise program.

Among the healthy foods are:

- Water – This should be the drink you use whenever you are thirsty. The kidneys use water to filter out toxins and to produce urine. And no, coffee does not count even if it is made with water.

- Fatty Fish – Salmon, tuna, and other cold-water fatty fish are high in Omega3 fatty acids. Since the body cannot make Omega3 fatty acids, these make a good outside source.

- Sweet Potatoes – Sweet potatoes contain vitamins and minerals as well as being rich in fiber. One such mineral is potassium which may help balance the levels of sodium in the body. However, if you have kidney disease, you may want to reduce the consumption of sweet potatoes.

- Dark Leafy Greens – Included in this list are spinach, kale, and chard. All of which contain a variety of vitamins and minerals. They also contain antioxidants. They do tend to be high in potassium which may not be suitable for people on dialysis or if you are on a restricted diet.

- Dark Berries – This would include raspberries, strawberries, and blueberries. These are a great source of antioxidants and nutrients.

- Apples – Apples contain an important fiber called pectin. There are certain risk factors for kidney damage such as blood sugar and cholesterol. Pectin may help reduce some of these risk factors.

There are also some foods you should avoid:

- Phosphorous-rich foods – Consuming too much phosphorous can put stress on the kidneys which may lead to long term kidney damage. Some foods that are high in phosphorous are:

  Meat
  Dairy products
  Most grains
  Legumes
  Nuts
  Fish

- Red Meat – There are some types of protein that are more difficult for the kidneys to process. Red meat is one of them. There has been some research that shows people who eat a lot of red meat have a higher risk for kidney damage than those who do not.

- Egg Yolks – Although eggs are a protein, the yolks contain high amounts of phosphorous. If you have kidney disease, you should only be using the egg whites. When the body uses protein, it turns it into waste which the kidneys must filter out.

As you can see your diet is important and quite complex. Some of the foods which are considered good for your overall diet are not good for you if you have trouble with your kidneys. Balance is the key to a healthy diet.

Again, talk to a licensed dietitian or doctor before you decide to change your diet.

In the next chapter, we will start working with the lungs.

CHAPTER 12

THE LUNG MASSAGE & MERIDIAN

In this chapter we are going to work on stimulating the energy in your lungs.

Your lungs are not just the organs of breath. They also keep you connected to the universe. In the universe there is a constant flow and exchange of life force energy. Every time you breathe in you bring part of the energy of the universe into yourself. When you exhale, you give a part of yourself back to the universe.

The lungs regulate the energy we absorb from the universe, and they distribute the energy through your body. They control breathing, distributing oxygen to the blood, and work with the heart to circulate the blood and energy in your body.

When you become sexually aroused, you can pump positive energy through your body by using deep and full breaths. Remember, to be sexually aroused the whole body needs to be alive and full of energy. This is the purpose of the lungs.

If your lung energy is weak or congested it will be difficult to feel aroused and excited. This can lead to depression which is one of the biggest causes of impotence.

To stimulate the lung energy, you need to massage the lung points.

The lung energy is stimulated by lightly knocking on the chest with a loose fist. This will result in the opening the rib cage as well as relaxing the diaphragm. This will be like the way you stimulated the kidneys, except you will knock using the finger side of the fist.

Knock just below the collar bone to activate the lung points and stimulate the lung meridian.

Using both hands, continue to knock on and across the chest for at least one minute. When you feel the buzzing and tingling in the chest area, take 2 or 3 long deep breaths and feel the lungs open and energize.

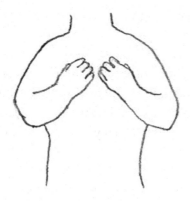

Now, let's talk about The Lung Meridian

The lung meridian begins deep in the solar plexus and runs downward, connecting with the large intestine. It then turns and winds up past the stomach and through the diaphragm. Here it divides and enters the lungs. It then reunites and runs up the middle of the windpipe to the throat, where it divides again.

It then surfaces near the front of the shoulder. From here, it goes down the front of the arm along the outer side of the bicep muscle. It continues down to the wrist toward the thumb, where it ends at the corner of the thumbnail.

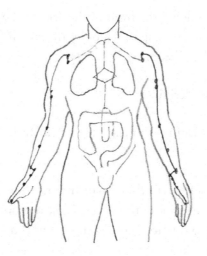

To balance the lung meridian:

Start with your hand on the opposite lung, i.e. your left hand on the right lung. Move your fingers outward to touch the first acupuncture point which is in the hollow near the front of the shoulder.

Follow the path of the meridian straight up. As you can see in the diagram, it only goes up a short distance. Then follow it down the front of the arm to the inside of the elbow.

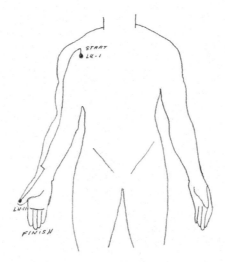

Trace the meridian down the front of the arm to the wrist at the base of the thumb. Continue tracing to the outer thumbnail where the meridian ends. Repeat for the other arm.

Flushing the Lung Meridian:

The first step in flushing is to trace the meridian in the reverse order of the natural flow.

Start from the outside of the thumbnail and trace up to the wrist and then the inner arm to the inside of the elbow. Continue up to the shoulder area and slightly down to the first acupuncture point (Lu 1) in the hollow near the front of the shoulder.

Then balance by tracing the meridian forward 3 times. Repeat this for the other arm.

In the next chapter we will start working with the liver and spleen.

CHAPTER 13

THE LIVER AND SPLEEN MASSAGE

In this chapter, you will be working with the liver and the spleen energy system.

The liver is about the size of a football and is located on your right side of the upper abdomen, tucked just behind the rib cage. You may remember that the liver's main job is to filter the blood from toxins and bacteria coming from the digestive tract, before passing it to the rest of the body.

The liver acts as the body's glucose (or fuel) reservoir and helps to keep your circulating blood sugar levels steady and constant. So, the proper functioning of the liver directly influences the regulation of sugar in the blood.

The liver plays a vital role in the strength of your erection because it transfers an exceptional amount of energy to the sexual center. You will not be able to relax if this energy is not flowing freely. If you can't relax, the energy can't flow. This means you will have a difficult time getting an erection even if you feel aroused.

Releasing the congestion in the liver and allowing your body to relax allows the liver energy to flow into your sexual center.

Now let's look at The Spleen

The spleen plays multiple roles that support the other organs in the body. One role is to act as a filter for blood as part of the immune system. The spleen manufactures our life-sustaining energy from food.

When the energy of the spleen is congested, it causes the mind to be overactive. This, in turn, causes worry and anxiety. The worry and anxiety make it difficult to be sexually aroused.

When the energy is flowing freely, you feel connected to yourself. When you are "connected to yourself", you can connect with others both sexually and emotionally.

The liver and the spleen are both located in the upper abdomen and the abdomen is the center of the body. When there is energy flowing in the abdomen it can flow to other parts of the body.

Let's see how you can stimulate the liver.

The liver is located on the right side of the upper abdomen.

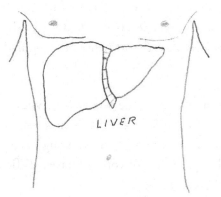

LIVER

First Place your right hand on the right side of the upper abdomen just below the rib cage. With your hand slightly cupped, so your entire hand is touching your body, gently press and massage the liver by rotating your hand in a circular, clockwise direction. Rotate at least 30 time.

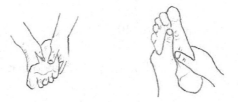

As you rotate your hand, use your power of visualization to see the energy moving from your hand into the liver. After you have completed at least 30 rotations, switch directions and do at least 30 rotations in a counter-clockwise direction.

The Liver Meridian

The liver meridian runs down the legs and into the feet. Massaging the feet will help stimulate the liver. Using both hands, massage each foot. Pay attention to the big toe and surrounding area because this is where the liver meridian ends. Spend at least 5 minutes massaging each foot to ensure that energy moves into the body.

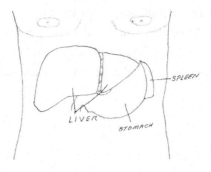

Now we will move on to Stimulating the Spleen

The spleen is located on the left side of the upper abdomen.

Place your left hand on the left side of your upper abdomen just below the rib cage. With your hand slightly cupped, so your entire hand is touching your body, gently press and massage the spleen by rotating your hand in a circular, clockwise direction for a minimum of 30 rotations.

As you rotate your hand, use your power of visualization to see the energy moving from your hand into the spleen. After the 30 rotations, switch directions and go at least 3o rotations in a counter-clockwise direction.

The spleen is associated with the earth element and the color yellow. The best way to recharge this energy is to reconnect it with the earth. This reconnection is best if done barefoot. Stand in an outside area such as your yard, garden, or anywhere you can be touching the ground.

Stand with your spine straight and your arms relaxed at your sides. Relax and feel the energy of the earth rising into your feet and up your legs. Visualize this in your mind. Feel and imagine a golden yellow light moving up your legs and filling your entire body. Feel the energy radiating throughout your belly.

Continue this meditation for 5 to 10 minutes.

Next, you will massage your abdomen

A light abdominal massage stimulates the circulation of the spleen energy. You can massage your abdomen from either a standing or sitting position as long as you keep your spine straight. Place your left palm on your upper abdomen and place your right palm on top of the left hand.

Breathing fully and gently, massage your abdomen with your palm moving in a clockwise direction. As you exhale, whisper the sound "huuuuuu". Continue the massage for at least 30 rotations and when you have finished them switch to a counter-clockwise direction for an additional 30 rotations.

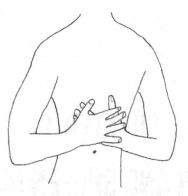

If you feel any tightness or congestion, using your fingertips <u>gently</u> work into the abdomen and try to feel any release. <u>This area is very sensitive so don't put a lot of pressure on it.</u> Remember to try to use deep full breaths and use your visualization power to send the energy into these organs.

Massaging the liver and the spleen will be a part of your regular exercise routine as you go through this book. Something to remember; these organs provide energy to your sexual center. Keeping the energy flowing freely in your abdomen is very important, so don't skimp on this part of your exercises.

In the next chapter, we will start working on the liver and spleen meridians.

CHAPTER 14

THE LIVER AND SPLEEN MERIDIANS

In this chapter, we will work on balancing your liver and spleen meridians.

First you will work on the liver meridian:

The liver meridian starts on the inside of the big toenail. It then goes across the top of the foot and passes in front of the inside ankle. From here it continues up along the inner side of the leg and thigh until it reaches the groin and pubic area. It then circles the genitals and enters the abdomen.

It then continues upward until it reaches the lower chest where it enters the liver and gall bladder. From here it turns internal and runs into the ribcage and up through the throat where it connects with the eyes. It ends at the crown of the head and connects with the governing channel.

As I mentioned before, the governing channel is one of the two major energy channels in your body and we will discuss it in detailing in an upcoming chapter.

One small branch of the meridian goes from the eyes downwards to the cheek where it curves around the inner surface of the lips.

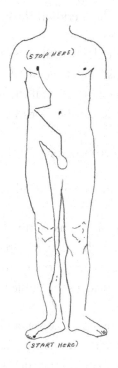

The meridian trace:

To trace the Liver Meridian, place the fingers at the inside base of the big toe (next to your second toe). Trace across the top of your foot and continue up the inside of the leg to the groin. Go around your genitals, and up the side of the ribcage to your first rib (which is in line with the breast directly under the nipple).

You can mentally trace the internal path which comes up the front of the chest to the chin, up the sides of the face to the center of the eyes, eyebrows, and up to the center of the forehead. From the forehead it moves to the top of your head.

As always, you can trace both sides together or do one side and then do the other.

W. R. Mills

The meridian flush:

To flush the meridian, trace the meridian backward one time starting at the point of your ribcage just under the nipple. Follow the pathway down the ribcage, around your genitals, and all the way down to the top of the foot. Continue to follow it across the foot to the inside of the big toe.

Follow this by tracing the pathway forward three times.

Next, we will look at the Spleen Meridian

The spleen meridian begins at the inside tip of the big toe and runs along the inside of the foot to the arch and turns up in front of the inner ankle. It then travels up the leg, just behind the bone along the inner side of the lower leg and thigh until it reaches the pubic bone.

From the pubic bone, it enters the lower abdomen, where it meets the conception vessel, the other main energy channel in the body. It then resurfaces briefly before penetrating the spleen and stomach.

The main channel then travels up through the diaphragm and over the chest, just outside the nipple. It continues up to the esophagus and ends under the tongue.

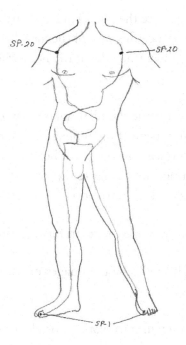

To trace the spleen meridian:

Start at the tip of the big toenail. Trace along the inside of the foot to the arch. Continue going up in front of the inner ankle and inner leg (just behind the bone). Continue up the inner thigh to the pubic bone.

The meridian in each leg then crisscrosses in the abdomen and continues up. It goes around the outside of the nipples to your collarbone, neck, and then ends under the tongue.

You can trace each side separately or at the same time.

To flush the meridian:

First, there are 2 forbidden points in Chinese medicine. I told you about the first one earlier. Never flush the heart meridian. The second one is: You rarely need to flush the spleen meridian.

To flush the meridian, trace the meridian backward one time, starting at the tip of the tongue. (Since this part of the meridian is internal, you can only trace it mentally.) Continue down the neck where it turns and goes toward your arm pits.

From here, you can trace the meridian physically to the collarbone and around the chest, just outside of the nipples. Crisscross the abdomen just above your naval and trace it to the pubic bone. Continue to trace down the inner part of the thigh all the way to the front of the inner ankle. From the ankle trace across the arch to the tip of the big toenail.

To complete the flush trace the meridian forward three times.

I realize this is complicated. Use the images provided to help follow the pathways.

In the next chapter you will start working on the heart meridian.

CHAPTER 15

THE HEART MASSAGE

In this chapter we will start working with the heart.

Many believe the heart is the king of all the organs. It is called this because it circulates blood and energy through your entire body. There is also a strong connection between the heart and your sexual center. The heart being the energy center of passion and affection rules over your entire being: the physical, emotional, mental, and even the subtle feelings you have.

Energy stuck in the heart is one of the biggest sexual problems we face. When the energy is not moving correctly, it is difficult to have deep feelings and connect with your partner.

Not communicating what is in your heart is the main reason the energy gets congested. As a result, negative emotions surface. In contrast, when you express what is in your heart, the energy is free to move.

The two strongest energies in your body are loving energy and sexual energy. Therefore, there is an intimate connection between your heart and your sexual center.

Fire is associated with the heart and it is this fire energy that brings about excitement and exhilaration. It is also what opens your sexual center.

To open the energy pathways of the heart you massage the chest.

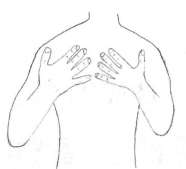

1) Massage the chest using your fingers, or knuckles if you need deeper pressure.

2) Look for tender areas along the sternum and between the ribs along the chest. Press into any tender areas gently, massaging them until you feel a release of the tenderness.

Spend some time massaging the sternum. This will release any emotional energy that has been congested in the heart center.

3) To end the massage, place your hands over your chest and project energy from your hands into the heart area.

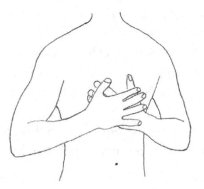

Visualize a bright red glow in your heart. Try to feel the connection between the heart and your sexual center.

Your tongue is the energetic extension of the heart. Exercising the tongue will help open the heart and your sexual energy because there is a very strong connection between the tongue, the heart, and your sexual energy.

Here are some exercises you can do for the tongue.

1) Bring the tip of the tongue in between your upper teeth and lips.

2) Circle the tongue down to the inside lower lips.

3) Continue this circle in front of the teeth and inside the lips for at least 30 complete rotations, then switch directions for an additional 30 rotations.

4) Vigorously massage the flat part of the tongue against the roof of your mouth at least 30 times.

This will generate heat through your head and your entire body. Feeling this heat is a good sign the heart and sexual center are opening. Massaging the tongue can have benefits to many of the organs in the body, as you can see from this illustration.

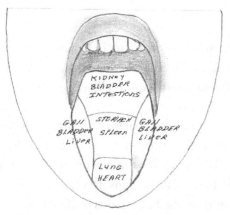

In the next chapter, you will work with the heart meridian.

CHAPTER 16

THE HEART MERIDIAN

"The heart is the sovereign of all organs and represents the consciousness of one's being. It is responsible for intelligence, wisdom, and spiritual transformation." The Chinese wrote this quote approximately 4,700 years ago.

The heart is much more than simply a physical structure that pumps 1.5 gallons of blood through your body each minute. It also produces hormones, has its own nervous system. It is the body's strongest electrical generator.

Many cultures consider the heart to be where love emanates as well as where our emotions are based and where the soul resides. There is much more to the heart; The heart is an intelligence system.

In 1991 Dr. Armour discovered that the heart had its own "little brain". Its name is the intrinsic cardiac nervous system. It has roughly 40,000 neurons that are like the neurons in the brain. This "little brain" carries information to the brain via the vagus nerve. In fact, the heart sends more signals to the brain than the brain sends to the heart.

It is the most intelligent system in the body. It has its own receptors and its own electromagnetic force. It is also the only force capable of changing our own DNA.

The hearts function dominates such things as:

Long-term memory

Thinking

Emotions

Intimacy

Cognition

Intelligence

Ideas

Sleep: if the Heart energy is strong a person will fall asleep easily and sleep soundly. If the heart energy is weak, the person's mind will "float," resulting in an inability to fall asleep. They may also have disturbed sleep or they may have excessive dreaming.

The heart is the King of all the organs. This means all your other organs will always sacrifice for your heart. They will give their energy to help your heart maintain balance. The up and down fluctuations of your emotions can damage your heart. That is why it is so important to keep your emotions in check.

The heart meridian is the energy channel for your heart. It has 3 branches. One branch goes from the heart down through the diaphragm where it swirls around the small intestine. Another branch extends through the throat to the eyes and to the tongue.

The third branch goes to the lungs and surfaces at the center of the armpit. From here the channel runs along the inner side of the forearm (the side opposite of the bicep). It then runs through the elbow to the wrist. From here it moves across the palm of your hand and ends at the tip of the little finger by the corner of the fingernail on the side toward the thumb.

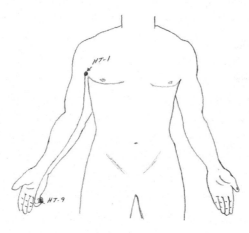

Although the heart meridian has its origins in the heart, it does not spread through the heart. Instead, it permeates the aorta and other major blood vessels entering and exiting the heart. It spreads throughout the major arteries and blood vessels and touches every part of your body. As you can see, keeping the heart meridian clear of congestion and blockages is crucial for your body.

Here are the steps to trace and balance the heart meridian:

1) Trace the heart meridian forward slowly using the palm of your hand. Start in the middle of the armpit and trace slowly along the inside lower edge of the arm, the side opposite your bicep muscle, to the elbow.

2) Follow this down your forearm to the palm of your hand.

3) Continue across the palm of your hand and end at the tip of the little finger as you squeeze both sides of the fingernail.

Repeat for the other arm.

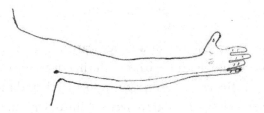

You can also mentally trace the inner 2 branches of the meridian, the one going up to the eyes and the one going down to the small intestine.

NEVER TRACE THE HEART MERIDIAN IN REVERSE.

You can trace the heart meridian as often as you wish. You can't overdo this tracing.

Here are some Extra Bonuses:

Rest one hand over your heart (the fourth chakra) and one hand on your tailbone (the second chakra or the sacral chakra). This will help the heart meridian and heart organ stay strong. Think of this as a relaxing meditation. I find this to be calming when used just before I fall asleep.

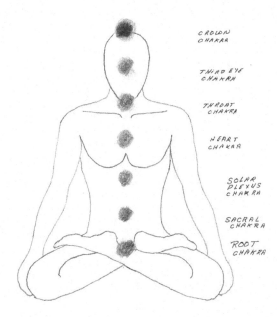

Second Bonus:

If you are feeling irregularity or a rapid heart rate, place both your little fingers in your mouth, with the back of the hands facing each other. Have one edge of your fingernail against the upper teeth and the other edge of the finger nail touching the bottom teeth. "Bite down" on the little finger. Hold this for at least 30 seconds to a minute. You are not trying to hurt yourself, so don't bite too hard.

This action sends energy directly into the heart meridian and removes it from the small intestine meridian.

Third Bonus:

This is the Shenmen or Spirit Door (or Gate) and it is on the palm side of the inner wrist directly down from the pinky finger. (It's acupuncture point HT-7.) Massage, this point for emotional issues and disconnection, especially related to sleep, insomnia, or "muddled" thinking. It helps relieve insomnia and anxiety. It also settles the spirit, calms the mind, and relieves confusion and anxiety.

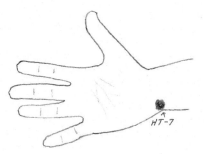

CHAPTER 17

RECAP

Before we close out part 3, I wanted to answer some questions I assume are going through your mind. Such as: If there are so many meridians running through my feet and legs, how do I know I am stimulating the correct one?

It is true that most of the meridians we are working with do run through your feet and legs, and it would be easy to get them confused.

Do you remember in the last lesson when I said your long-term memory, thinking, emotions, intelligence, and ideas are all dominated by the function of the heart? I also said your heart is an intelligence system. It is in fact the most intelligent system in your body.

So, when you are tracing or flushing a meridian, you must have a <u>clear intent</u> on which one you are working with and <u>why you are working with it</u>. If you keep a clear picture of this, your heart and your brain will keep everything on course. Always keep in mind the power of your heart and you won't go wrong.

You have now been through parts 1, 2, and 3. So you have accomplished three of your goals so far. You accomplished these goals because they were realistic. Each step you take on this journey, climbing this mountain, is one step closer to achieving the victory you so desperately want.

You have learned a lot of things. You have learned that your bodily organs are all connected. There are certain organs that have a direct connection to your sexual center.

You have learned there are meridians, or energy channels, running through your body. You have also learned that these channels can become congested and obstruct the flow of your life energy.

You have learned, or at least you are working on, how visualization can directly influence your body and your entire life. You have learned how top professionals and athletes use their power of visualization to achieve their goals and how this same power is available to you. Use this power every day and your life will change drastically.

Before we move on to part 4, I want to tell you a quick story about one of my experiences and visualization.

I had a co-worker who made my life miserable. I heard about the power of visualization and how I could use it to overcome my deep anger toward him. Every morning and night I visualized watching the two of us laughing and talking like we were old friends. I did this as a third person not as a participant, so all I could do was observe.

Every day I watched the two of us getting along and having fun. One day, I noticed that I didn't have the animosity toward him anymore. We became friends <u>and</u> I didn't have the same experiences at work as I did before. There truly is great power in visualization and it is yours to use.

In the next chapter, we are going to start part two of the Penis Enhancement Qigong series.

PART 4

THE SECRET OF SOUNDS

CHAPTER 18

THE LUNG SOUND

In this chapter, I will introduce you to the Healing Sounds

In the part 3, we went through the 5 major organs of the body associated with your sexual energy.

There are specific <u>sounds</u> you can make as you exhale that can help cleanse, heal, and put you in touch with these specific organs.

There is also a sixth sound, called The Triple Warmer. It is not associated with an organ. Instead, it is composed of three regions of the body, the upper, the middle, and the lower. The sixth sound balances these three regions of your body.

Each of the 5 organs related to the meridians is also associated with an element.

There are 5 elements:

- Wood
- Metal
- Water
- Fire
- Earth

In addition, each organ is associated with a specific color. Visualizing the organ surrounded by its color as you exhale while making the corresponding sound helps the process of cleansing, healing, and getting in touch with these organs.

The lungs are associated with the element metal, the sound S-s-s-s-s-s, and the color white.

The Kidneys are associated with the element water, the sound Ch-u-w-a-a-y, and the color blue.

The Liver is associated with the element wood, the sound Sh-h-h-h-h-h, and the color green.

The Heart is associated with the element fire, the sound H-a-w-w-w-w, and the color Red.

The Spleen is associated with the element Earth, the sound Wh-o-o-o-o, and the color yellow.

The Triple Warmer is Not associated with any element. It is, however, associated with the sound H-e-e-e-e. There is no color associated with the triple warmer.

The first sound I would like to work with is for the Lungs. As you recall, the lungs are the organs of breath and allow us to take in and connect with a part of the universe every time we breathe in and out. Your breathing pumps energy throughout your entire body.

Here are the steps for making the <u>Lung Sound</u>:

1) Mentally place your awareness (concentrate) on your lungs.

2) Take a deep abdominal breath.

3) Visualize your lungs bathed in white light.

4) Close your mouth so that your teeth are just touching and keep your lips slightly open.

5) Place the tip of your tongue against your lower gums just below your bottom front teeth.

6) Exhale and very gently make the sound S-s-s-s-s-s-s-s

7) Try to feel the heat radiating out of your lungs.

8) Repeat at least 3 times.

In the next series of chapters, we will work through the rest of the healing sounds and how to use them.

CHAPTER 19

THE KIDNEY & LIVER SOUNDS

This chapter will focus on The Kidney and Liver Sounds.

Remember, your kidneys are vital to you having an abundance of sexual energy.

Organ	Element	Sound	Color
Kidneys	Water	Ch-u-w-a-a-y	Blue

Here are the steps for The Kidney Sound:

1) Place your awareness (concentrate) on both the left and right kidneys.

2) Take a deep abdominal breath. Visualize both kidneys bathed in a blue light (like sapphire).

3) Exhale slowly and quietly make the healing sound Ch-u-w-a-a-a (long A sound), as you pull in your abdomen. Feel the heat radiating out of your kidneys.

Repeat at least 3 times.

Since the kidneys are associated with the water element and this is usually associated with cold water, you may feel excess cold radiating from your kidneys instead of heat while doing the kidney sound.

Next, let's go over the liver sound.

The liver also transfers an exceptional amount of energy to your sexual center and plays a vital role in the strength of your erection.

Organ	Element	Sound	Color
Liver	Wood	Sh-h-h-h-h	Green

Here are the steps for the Liver Sound:

1) Place your awareness (concentrate) on your liver.

2) Take a deep abdominal breath.

3) Visualize your liver bathed in Emerald-Green light.

4) Exhale and quietly make the healing sound Sh-h-h-h-h-h-

5) Feel the heat radiating out of your liver.

Repeat this at least 3 times.

In the next chapter you will continue to work on the next healing sounds.

CHAPTER 20

THE HEART & SPLEEN SOUNDS

We will start this chapter, with the heart sound.

Remember, your heart has a strong connection to your sexual center. It is the energy center of passion and affection.

Organ	Element	Sound	Color
Heart	Fire	H-a-w-w-w	Red

Here are the steps for the heart healing sound:

1) Place your awareness (concentrate) on your heart.

2) Take a deep abdominal breath.

3) Visualize your heart bathed in a bright red light.

4) Round your lips, open your mouth slightly, exhale, and make the healing sound H-a-w-w-w.

5) Feel the heat being expelled from your heart.

Repeat at least 3 times.

Next, let's go over the Spleen sound.

Congestion in the spleen energy causes the mind to be overactive which can cause worry and anxiety.

Organ	Element	Sound	Color
Spleen	Earth	Wh-o-o-o-o	Yellow

Here are the steps for the Spleen Healing Sound:

1) Place your awareness (concentrate) on your spleen.

2) Take a deep abdominal breath.

3) Visualize your spleen bathed in a bright yellow light.

4) Let your lips form a small circle and exhale slowly as you quietly make the healing sound Wh-o-o-o-o

Repeat at least 3 times.

In the next chapter we will go over the Triple Warmer.

CHAPTER 21

THE TRIPLE WARMER SOUND

In this chapter we will cover The Triple Warmer Sound.

The triple warmer sound will help balance the upper, middle, and lower body sections.

Organ	Element	Sound	Color
Triple Warmer	------	H-e-e-e-e	----

Here are the steps for the triple warmer healing sound:

1) Take a deep abdominal breath.

2) The triple warmer does not have a color associated with it for you to visualize. Instead, as you exhale visualize a wave (like an ocean wave) moving down your body starting from your head.

See the wave going down your chest, solar plexus, and through your lower abdomen.

3) Exhale slowly and as quietly as you can make the healing sound H-e-e-e-e-e-e

4) Feel heat moving down with the wave and out of your body as you make the healing sound. (You might feel it exit the body through your fingertips or toes.)

I realize these last few chapters have gone by quickly, but do not underestimate the importance of these exercises. These will not only help you get in touch with the organs that control your sexual energy, they will also help heal any energy blockages in the organs.

Continue to do these exercises as part of your routine.

You made it through part 4 and you have learned a lot.

So far it seems all you have done is biology and anatomy. Although it may seem boring, you need to have the basics of this in place so we can start working with making changes in your sexual energy.

Keep working on everything you have learned up to this point and it will start making more sense from here on out. We will start pulling this together in the coming sections.

In the next part, we will cover the pelvic floor, and then we will look at the prostate. After that we will start working on some exercises to bring this all into focus.

PART 5

THE PELVIC FLOOR

CHAPTER 22

THE PELVIC FLOOR & YOUR SEXUAL ENERGY

In this chapter we will discuss the Pelvic Floor and how it relates to your sexual energy. Perhaps I have lived a sheltered life, but I had never heard of the term "Pelvic Floor". I knew where all the external parts were, but I never considered the internal muscles that controlled them.

The pelvic floor is a group of muscles that sit, like a trampoline, within your pelvis. In the front these muscles attach to the pubic bone. They attach to the tailbone (coccyx) in the back and from each sitting bone on the sides.

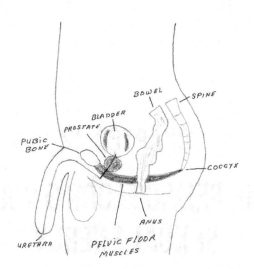

These muscles work 24 - hours a day to support your bladder, colon, rectum, and sexual organs. I used the reference of a trampoline because these muscles can move up and down as they support the organs in the pelvic area.

The pelvic floor muscles do more than support the organs. They also help your bladder and rectum relax and contract when necessary. These are the same muscles you use when you try not to pee or pass gas. These muscles also contract when you are having sex.

The pelvic floor muscles have 5 main functions:

- Support Function: The pelvic floor muscles act as a basket to support our pelvic organs (bladder and rectum) against increases in abdominal pressure.

- Sphincter Function: The muscles of the pelvic floor wrap around and control the opening of your bladder and rectum. When there is an increase in abdominal pressure (when you cough, sneeze, laugh or jump) these muscles contract around your urethra and anus to prevent leakage.

Equally as important, these muscles must relax and lengthen to allow you to urinate or have bowel movements easily.

- Stability Function: Because of their attachments to the pelvis and hips, these muscles assist other muscles in your abdomen, hip, and back to control the movement of your hip joints.

- Sexual Function: During intercourse, the pelvic floor muscles help to achieve and sustain your erection. Having strong pelvic floor muscles is necessary for having an orgasm. Excessive tension or sensitivity of the pelvic floor can also contribute to pain during or after intercourse.

- Sump-pump Function: The calf muscles in your leg act to pump blood and lymphatic fluid back up towards your heart. The pelvic floor muscles act as a blood/lymph pump for the pelvis.

When your pelvic muscles are too loose, or too tight, problems can occur. Weak or damaged pelvic floor muscles can lead to urinary leakage, accidental bowel leakage, and pelvic organ prolapse. This is a condition in which the rectum or bladder can bulge or drop completely out of the body. This is more common in women, but it can also occur in men.

If these muscles are too tight it can be hard to relax causing difficult bowel movements. This can also cause incomplete bladder emptying and burning during urination. Tight muscles can cause a weak urinary stream, constipation, or pain when having sex.

Like any other muscle in your body, pelvic floor muscles are controllable and trainable through physical therapy. We will be starting that training in the next chapter.

You may be wondering what the pelvic floor has to do with your sexual energy. As I mentioned earlier, there are energy centers located in different parts of your body. There are 7 major energy centers called chakras.

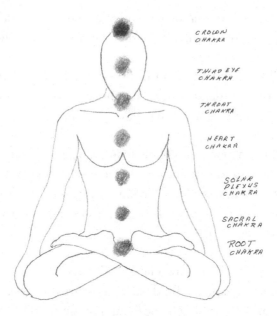

CROWN
CHAKRA

THIRD EYE
CHAKRA

THROAT
CHAKRA

HEART
CHAKRA

SOLAR
PLEXUS
CHAKRA

SACRAL
CHAKRA

ROOT
CHAKRA

There is one fundamental chakra called the root chakra and it is located at the end of your tailbone. (This is your sexual energy center.) The back of the pelvic floor muscles also attach to the end of the tailbone. By starting with the energy center that is in your sexual center we will be laying the foundation for working with the other six energy centers.

Your Root Chakra links to your sex muscles. The stronger your root the easier it will be for you to control and direct your sexual energy.

When we talked earlier about the different organs associated with the energy centers I talked about blocked or congested energy. When these energy centers are all open and energy is flowing freely, your body and mind are optimized for success both in and out the bedroom.

If there is an imbalance in the root chakra it will throw your whole system out of whack. Energy rises from the root chakra up to the second chakra (sacral or sexual chakra). Thus, it is the root chakra that determines how much energy you have.

If you have little energy, you won't be able to last long in bed. Having a strong root gives you stamina and endurance that allows your body to keep going. As you can see, your Root Chakra is essential for a healthy and satisfying sex life.

Men in general have a weaker Root Chakra than women and it is often the reason for a weak or no erection. Your body needs the energy to pump all that blood needed for sex.

In the next chapter, we will discuss restoring your sexual energy.

CHAPTER 23

RESTORING YOUR SEXUAL ENERGY

In this chapter we will be discussing how you can restore your sexual energy.

Many people believe you waste your sexual energy every time you ejaculate unless it is for reproduction.

Remember, I told you your body only uses your greatest of energy for your sperm. Ejaculating depletes your source of vital energy instead of allowing it to spread to the rest of the body.

I know what you are thinking. What fun is sex if you don't ejaculate? What you are going to learn in this book is going to blow your mind. You can have an orgasm or multiple orgasms without ejaculating.

But first things first.

Regulating and controlling your ejaculation does not mean becoming celibate. In fact, it is just the opposite. As you know, almost immediately upon ejaculation your penis gets soft, and you are pretty much finished.

Now I want you to imagine how it will be when you have all the experiences of ejaculation without ejaculating. Your erection will remain hard and you can keep going until you decide to ejaculate.

No longer will your partner complain that you went too quickly and she didn't get to finish. You will definitely be her "man of steel".

So, let's go over how you can make this happen.

You have a set of muscles in your pelvic floor called the Pubococcygeus Muscles I am going to call them the PC Muscles for short.

They run from the pubic bone in the front all the way to the tailbone in the back.

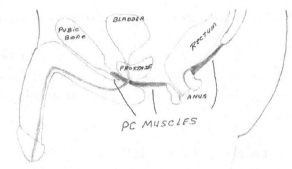

Let's look at how to exercise your PC Muscles.

Exercising your PC muscle will enable you to develop the ability to control your ejaculation. Doing these exercises will also improve urinary flow and increase blood circulation, which will also enhance your penis size and sensation.

Exercising the PC muscles will also improve your stamina and give you the ability to have multiple orgasms. As a bonus, this will also improve the health of your prostate, which we will cover in the next part of the book.

The first step is locating your PC muscle. You have probably known its location for years and didn't realize it. If you can make your penis move on its own when you have an erection, you know where the PC muscle is.

If you are unable to do this, the next time you are urinating try to stop the urine flow. The muscle you used to stop the flow is the PC muscle.

After you have identified the PC muscle, don't make it a habit to stop your urination when you are going to the bathroom. This can cause you more problems than it will help.

To help you focus on the muscle, I want you to try to flex this muscle and see if you can do it somewhere between 10 and 20 times. Take a break right now and see if you can flex it 20 times.

If your PC muscle feels tired after doing the 20 flexes it is out of shape.

You will notice that the PC muscle goes all the way back to the tailbone. Stopping the flow of urine uses the front part of the muscle. When you are trying not to pass gas by contracting your anus, you are using the middle part of the muscle.

The difficult part of doing a PC muscle flex is using the back part of the muscle. You must learn to use this part of the muscle. This is at the heart of your sexual energy center.

When you are using the back part of the muscle, your tailbone will move. Concentrate on pulling the back part of the muscle up until you can lift the tailbone.

Moving the tailbone will require a lot more work than simply cutting off the flow of urine, which is what you have been doing.

The strength or your ejaculation, your erectile strength and firmness, and your prostate health are all influenced by how often you perform these PC exercises. I want you to aim for at least 200 up to 500 per day.

With practice, you will be able to hold off the urge to ejaculate just by squeezing your PC muscle as tight as you can.

Here are the PC Muscle exercises.

These exercises can be done while you are sitting, standing, lying down, or on hands and knees like a baby crawling. One of the most common ways a person starts is by lying on the floor with your knees up and apart while your feet are flat on the floor and your hands at your sides.

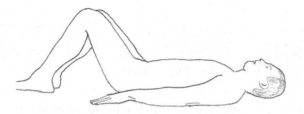

But any of these methods will work. Try these various positions and see which one feels the most comfortable for you.

You will also use visualization with these exercises. When you are doing the exercises, close your eyes and get a good visual picture of your sexual organs in your mind. Every time you do a PC flex, visualize your penis growing a little bit and becoming the size you want it to be. Also visualize your PC muscles getting stronger. Focus on every flex, while you are visualizing its effect.

You will start the exercise with the Warmup:

Start out by squeezing and relaxing your PC muscle at a consistent pace for 30 flexes. At the same time, as you flex, try to lift the back of the muscle up towards your spine. It is the flexing and lifting together that strengthens the muscle.

At the end of the 30 flexes, rest for 30 seconds. Then continue to do 2 more sets.

After the warmup, there will be an increase in blood flow and sexual energy. This will help give you better control over your PC muscle.

Now you are ready for the PC Clamps:

PC Clamps are done by quickly squeezing and releasing the PC muscle. Start with 30 PC clamps and build up to 100 or more. Eventually build up to at least 300 PC clamps a day and do the exercise every other day. The latest studies have shown that these are more effective if you do them every other day instead of every day.

You might not be able to follow the warm-up with 30 PC Clamps until your PC Muscle is stronger. It's okay not to be able to do this many. It takes time to build up to this. Don't rush it.

You are going to find out that you will <u>want</u> to continue these exercises for the rest of your life. The PC muscle heals and reacts quickly. As a result, you may find yourself waking up with a hard erection almost every morning.

When you can easily do the warmup and PC Clamps, continue to the next exercise.

Here are the steps for the next exercise:

The Long Squeeze:

First, warm-up with 30 PC clamps, then flex as hard and as deep as you can. When you can't squeeze any deeper, hold the squeeze where you are for 20 seconds.

Rest for 30 seconds, then repeat 5 times.

Again, this will take time to build up the strength of the PC muscle to do these. Don't rush it.

Everyone is different, but after a month or two, you should be able to squeeze and hold for at least a minute at a time. Work your way up to 10 sets of 2-minute-long holds.

Performing this exercise will give you erections of steel and the ability to last as long as you desire in bed.

I have given you a lot in the last part of this chapter. Don't try to do as many as I have stated for your goal right off the bat. Work your way up to these numbers. Your PC muscle is not ready for you to bombard it with this much work. Build this muscle slowly like you would any other muscle.

Doing these exercises every other day will give the muscle time to rest and strengthen between exercises.

In the next chapter, we will start you on an exercise to strengthen your core.

CHAPTER 24

THE CORE WORKOUT

In this chapter I am going to share some exercises with you that will not only help you please your partner but will also generally keep you healthy.

There is scientific evidence that exercising on a regular basis can improve your sexual function. Men who exercise more often are less likely to suffer from sexual dysfunctions.

While exercising regularly is a good place to start, there are some exercises that are better than others for sexual health and performance. The first one is Cardio-vascular. The last thing you want is to be gasping for air in the middle of making love.

An easy cardio-vascular exercise is simply walking. Start slowly and build up to a brisk pace or even a jog. Be mindful of your knees and ankles. A jog might be too much for them. I have arthritis in my feet and jogging would not be good for me.

You can also use an elliptical at the gym, or go for a hike or even take a swim. Anything that gets and keeps your heart rate up for an extended period works. (If you have ever suffered from a heart attack, the doctor will put you on a walking exercise.) Pick an activity that you enjoy so you will stick with it regularly.

Another set of exercises that will transform your sexual energy are Core Exercises. When you're trying to please your partner, a weak core could lead to exhaustion before either partner has finished. When I talk about your core, I am talking about all the muscles in your midsection.

Here is the first exercise. It's called The Plank.

The plank is simple to perform and it is paramount for good health, which includes your sexual health. It builds muscles around your abs, back, and pelvis, all of which can make a difference in lasting longer in bed.

Lie on your stomach with your palms down about shoulder-width apart under your shoulders. This is the position you would be in if you were doing a pushup.

Keeping your back as straight as possible, use your hands and arms to push your body up. The only parts that are touching the floor are your hands and your toes. You can use your forearms to hold yourself up if it is not comfortable using your hands. You can also use your knees if it is too difficult to stay up on your toes.

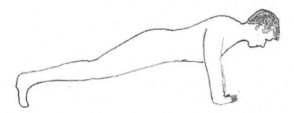

Hold this position for approximately one minute if you can. Don't force yourself to last that long. Work up to one minute if you need to.

This next exercise will continue what you are building with the plank. It is the Side Plank. Doing side planks will ensure you are hitting the rest of the abdominal muscles, especially the muscles along your sides.

Side planks are not as easy to do as regular planks. They take more practice and more balance. You Perform a side plank by <u>lying</u> on your side and raising yourself up onto your elbow, keeping your hip off the floor and your legs either stacked or staggered.

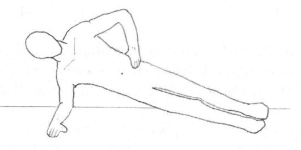

Position Your shoulder directly above your elbow, and your body should be in a straight line. When you have mastered this, raise your body further up by coming off your elbow and onto your hand. Doing this is more difficult than doing the first part of the side plank exercise.

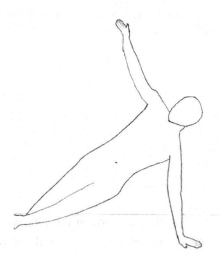

Breathe and hold for several seconds before switching sides.

Next, we have the gluteal bridge. The bridge not only works the muscles in the pelvic floor, but it can also help your hamstrings and glutes so you can thrust better, providing more pleasure for yourself and your lover.

Lie on the floor, or mat, knees bent and feet on the ground. Your palms should be on the floor next to your sides. Focus on your core as you push through your heels and raise your pelvis off the ground.

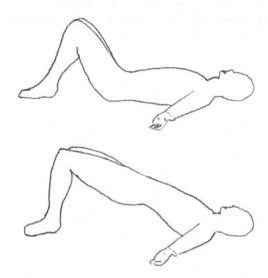

Make sure your shoulders and upper-back stay on the floor. When you reach a stiff bridge at the top, hold that position and squeeze your glutes (butt muscles).

Hold this until you feel your muscles tire. Release your glutes and lower back to the floor.

Working on your core by doing these simple exercises, will give you better overall health as well as improve your sex drive.

This brings us to the end of another section of the book.

By completing this section, you have reached another goal in your process to enhance your sexual life and energy. It is important that you keep these small goals in your mind and that you continue to visualize the result you are obtaining.

Continue to do the exercises that we have already gone through.

Keep in mind they will work if you continue to do them.

If you must miss a day, the world is not going to end, and all is not in vain. Simply pick them back up the next day but try not to miss any scheduled days. Missing days will only take a longer time for the process to work.

CHAPTER 25

ADVANCED KEGEL EXERCISES

As always, before you undertake any exercise routine, consult your doctor and make sure you can safely perform the exercises.

Kegel exercises will strengthen the muscles of the pelvic floor. In the previous chapters you learned how to perform Kegel exercises. This chapter provides you with an alternative method of performing the same exercises.

The methods presented here are more difficult to perform but you might find these methods more valuable.

There are 2 stages in achieving and maintaining an erection. The first stage is the vascular stage in which blood flows to the penis. The second stage is the muscular stage, and this is the stage of maintaining the erection and reaching ejaculation.

There are 2 specific muscles in the pelvic floor that are responsible for achieving and maintaining the erection. These muscles are the Bulbocavernosus Muscle and the Ischiocavernosus Muscle.

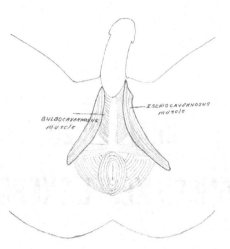

The Bulbocavernosus muscle is responsible for the formation of the erection and the Ischiocavernosus muscle maintains the blood pressure in the penis. These muscles working together bring about the orgasm.

Controlling the contraction of these muscles can increase the duration of the erection and possibly delay the ejaculation. The intensity of the orgasm is dependent on your ability to control these muscles.

In these exercises you will work on each muscle in two ways, strength and stamina. The strengthening of the muscles will increase your ability to contract them while the stamina will increase the ability of the muscle to stay clinched over time.

These exercises will allow you to improve the strength and stamina of the muscles while performing physical (sexual) activity. Since you will be using these muscles while in the act of sexual intercourse, it makes sense to practice them while performing the same actions you will be using while having sex.

Performing these contraction exercises while training the muscles used for traditional sexual positions will give you real-world experience. In the previous chapters you performed these exercises while sitting or standing, now you will perform the exercises in the relevant sexual positions.

The pelvic tilt

There are 4 muscle groups that control the pelvis movement. They are:

The Erector Spinae muscles. These are the muscles along the spine.

The Abdominal muscles. These are the muscles along the front of the abdomen.

The Hamstring muscles. These muscles are around and above the knee.

The Hip Flexor muscles. These muscles are found in your hips and along the lower spine.

These 4 groups of muscles are the muscles you use when you thrust your hips during sex. The erector spinae muscles and the hip flexor muscles work together when you thrust your hips forward. The abdominal muscles and the hamstring muscles work together when you thrust your hips backwards.

You will be using these muscle groups in your exercises to strengthen these core muscles. This will provide the foundation for the movements you use when having sexual intercourse.

Exercise positions

During these exercises you will use the positions you are most likely to use when having sexual intercourse. The first position will be with you lying in the plank position using your elbows or hands to support you as you would in the missionary position.

The second position will be lying on your back as you would if your partner were on the top (commonly called the cowgirl position).

W. R. Mills

The third position will be with you kneeling on one or two knees as you would in the doggie-style position.

Be careful when you start these exercises. Do not try to start these exercises vigorously. Start slowly and build up your endurance.

In the next chapter you will do exercise position 1.

CHAPTER 26

ADVANCED KEGEL EXERCISE 1

As mentioned, you previously did Kegel exercises from a standing or sitting position. Now you will perform them in the bed. Performing them in bed will allow you to train your body in the positions and surroundings you use when having sex. The soft surface will also help strengthen the muscles better than a hard surface.

When performing the exercises do not hold your breath, instead try to breathe as normally as possible. Hopefully by now your normal breathing will be abdominal breathing.

More than likely, you have not tried to do Kegel exercises from these positions, so they may feel awkward at first. But these are the positions you will be in while having sexual intercourse.

As with any exercise you may not be able to maintain the exercise for the required time. This is not unusual, and you will be able to increase the time as you continue.

When doing these exercises, you will be contracting the PC muscles for 5 seconds followed by 5 seconds of rest. As time goes forward and your PC muscle gets stronger, you can increase the length of time you contract the muscle from 5 seconds to 10 seconds. After a while you should be able to increase the contraction to 15 seconds.

Position 1 – The Missionary Position:

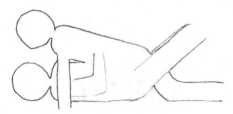

Exercise 1:

The missionary position is one of the most common sexual positions. The man is on top with his partner under him. Doing these exercises with you in the plank position will help strengthen the muscles used for missionary type sex.

You have used this position before when you were doing the core exercises. The exercises using the missionary position will work the muscles in the abdomen as well as the hip flexor and shoulder muscles.

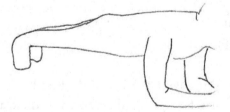

Lie in the plank position with your toes and forearms resting on the bed. Tilt your pelvis forward and backwards using a rate you find comfortable.

Start by tilting your pelvis for 30 seconds followed by a 30 second rest. Repeat 2 times.

As your muscles get stronger, increase the time from 30 seconds to 45 seconds. Repeat 2 times.

Slowly increase the time to 60 seconds. Repeat 2 times.

Tilting Your Pelvis

Tilting your pelvis is not moving your hips up and down. In Chapter 2 (Your Breathing and Posture) you learned how to tilt your pelvis. Think of your hips as swiveling on a ball joint.

When you tilt your hips, you are really pulling your pelvic bone up or pushing it down. These are not large sweeping movements. You are training and exercising muscles.

When you are tilting forward you will be tightening your abdominal muscles and tilting your pelvis toward your front. When you are pulling out, you are tilting your pelvis back and your butt moves up slightly. These subtle movements will take time for you to become accustomed to, so give yourself time.

Exercise 2:

Lie in the plank position as you did in exercise 1 with your toes and forearms resting on the bed. Keeping your body as straight as possible, slide your shoulder blades apart and then together. You learned how to do this in Chapter 2 (Breathing and Posture).

With your toes and forearms being the only part of your body touching the bed you will feel more pressure on your back and shoulder blades. Don't try to rush this. Take your time learning how to perform this exercise.

Continue to move your shoulder blades in and out while performing the rest of the exercise.

When you are first starting, and you are moving the shoulder blades, contract the PC muscle and hold this contraction for 5 seconds. Follow this by resting the PC muscle for 5 seconds. Do not stop moving your shoulder blades in and out during the 5 second rest cycle. Continue this repetition for 30 seconds.

W. R. Mills

(In Chapter 23 (Restoring Your Sexual Energy) you learned how to contract the PC muscle and you also worked on holding the contraction for several seconds.)

After 30 seconds, stop everything and rest for 30 seconds. Repeat this process 2 more times.

As your muscles get stronger you can increase the time you are holding the contraction of the PC muscle from 5 seconds to 10 seconds. You can also increase the duration of the exercise from 30 seconds to 45 seconds. Repeat this process 2 more times.

Work your way up until you are holding the contraction of the PC muscle to 15 seconds followed by a 5 second rest. Continue this repetition for 60 seconds. After 60 seconds, stop everything and rest for 30 seconds. Repeat 2 times.

CHAPTER 27

ADVANCED KEGELS EXERCISE 2

As always, before you undertake any exercise routine, consult your doctor, and make sure you can safely perform the exercises.

You will perform this exercise in the bed. Performing them in bed will allow you to train your body in the positions and surroundings you use when having sex. The soft surface will also help strengthen the muscles better than a hard surface.

When performing the exercises do not hold your breath, instead try to breathe as normally as possible. Hopefully by now your normal breathing will be abdominal breathing.

When doing these exercises, you will be contracting the PC muscles for 5 seconds followed by 5 seconds of rest. As time goes forward and your PC muscle gets stronger, you can increase the length of time you contract the muscle from 5 seconds to 10 seconds. After a while you should be able to increase the contraction to 15 seconds.

As with any exercise you may not be able to maintain the exercise for the required time. This is not unusual, and you will be able to increase the time as you continue.

Position 2 – The Cowgirl Position

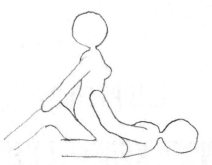

This is the easiest position as you simply need to lie on your back with your knees bent upward. The only challenge you will have is your ability to tilt your pelvis and slightly raise your hips. This will help strengthen the knee and hip extensors and the erector spinae muscles.

Once you start the exercise continue to tilt your pelvis throughout the duration of it. You will also be contracting and holding the contraction of the PC muscle for a set amount of time.

As an example, when you start the exercise, you will start tilting your pelvis up and down. While you are doing this, you will also contract the PC muscle and hold the contraction for the required number of seconds. You will continue to tilt your pelvis while you rest the PC muscle for 5 seconds. This means your pelvis will continue to move during the entire duration of the exercise.

Exercise 1:

Lie on your back with your knees bent upward so the flat of your feet are touching the bed. Tilt your pelvis up and down at a pace that feels comfortable.

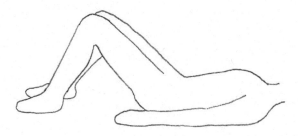

Start slowly. Tilt your pelvis (up and down) and contract your PC muscle. Hold the contraction for 5 seconds. Continue to tilt your pelvis while you rest the PC muscle for 5 seconds.

Continue this cycle of contracting and resting for 30 seconds (while you continue to tilt your pelvis). Then stop everything and rest for 30 seconds. Repeat 2 times.

As your muscles get stronger, increase the time of the contraction from 5 seconds to 10 seconds. Continue this cycle of contracting and resting for 45 seconds (while you continue to tilt your pelvis). Stop everything and rest for 30 seconds. Repeat 2 times.

Work your way up until you can contract and hold the PC muscle for 15 seconds. Continue to tilt your pelvis while you rest the PC muscle for 5 seconds.

Continue this cycle of contracting and resting for 60 seconds (while you continue to tilt your pelvis). Stop everything and rest for 30 seconds. Repeat 2 times.

Exercise 2:

Lie on your back with your knees bent upward so the flat of your feet are touching the bed. Lift your pelvis up and down at a comfortable pace. Again, the movement of lifting your pelvis off the bed is a continuous motion regardless of the flexing of the PC muscle.

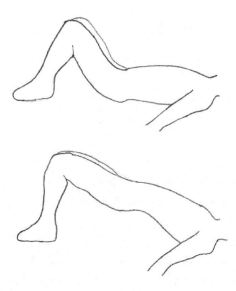

Again, start slowly. Lift your pelvis up and down off the bed and contract your PC muscle. Hold the contraction for 5 seconds. While you continue lifting and lowering your pelvis from the bed rest your PC muscle for 5 seconds. Continue this complete cycle for 30 seconds. Stop everything and rest for 30 seconds. Repeat 2 times.

As your muscles get stronger, increase the time you are holding the contraction from 5 seconds to 10 seconds. While you continue lifting and lowering your pelvis from the bed, rest your PC muscle for 5 seconds. Continue this complete cycle for 45 seconds. Stop everything and rest for 30 seconds. Repeat 2 times.

Work your way up until you can hold the contraction for 15 seconds. While you continue lifting and lowering your pelvis from the bed, rest your PC muscle for 5 seconds. Continue this complete cycle for 60 seconds. Stop everything and rest for 30 seconds. Repeat 2 times.

Exercise 3:

In this exercise you will lie flat on your back. You will raise and lower your hips while contracting your PC muscle and holding the contraction for the specified time. To raise your hips off the bed, push down with your heels.

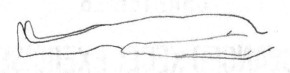

Start slowly. Lift your pelvis up and down off the bed and contract your PC muscle. Hold the contraction for 5 seconds. While you continue lifting and lowering your pelvis from the bed, rest your PC muscle for 5 seconds. Continue this complete cycle for 30 seconds. Stop everything and rest for 30 seconds. Repeat 2 times.

As you get stronger, increase the time you are holding the contraction from 5 seconds to 10 seconds. While you continue lifting and lowering your pelvis from the bed, rest your PC muscle for 5 seconds. Continue this complete cycle for 45 seconds. Stop everything and rest for 30 seconds. Repeat 2 times.

Work your way up until you can hold the contraction for 15 seconds. While you continue lifting and lowering your pelvis from the bed, rest your PC muscle for 5 seconds. Continue this complete cycle for 60 seconds. Stop everything and rest for 30 seconds. Repeat 2 times.

CHAPTER 28

ADVANCED KEGEL EXERCISE 3

As always, before you undertake any exercise routine, consult your doctor and make sure you can safely perform the exercises.

Additional Emphasis

You will perform this exercise in the bed. Performing them in bed will allow you to train your body in the positions and surroundings you use when having sex. The soft surface will also help strengthen the muscles better than a hard surface.

When performing the exercises do not hold your breath, instead try to breathe as normally as possible. Hopefully by now your normal breathing will be abdominal breathing.

When doing these exercises, you will be contracting the PC muscles for 5 seconds followed by 5 seconds of rest. As time goes forward and your PC muscle gets stronger, you can increase the length of time you contract the muscle from 5 seconds to 10 seconds. After a while you should be able to increase the contraction to 15 seconds.

As with any exercise you may not be able to maintain the exercise for the required time. This is not unusual, and you will be able to increase the time as you continue.

Position 3 – Doggie Position

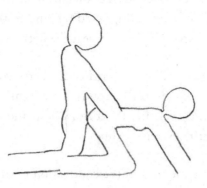

This position will be a little more challenging than the previous positions. As you can see in the illustration you usually have your partner to hold on to while making love. When you are doing the exercises, you will be balancing on your knees and toes with no one to hold on to. These exercises will use all the muscle groups previously mentioned to keep your balance.

Exercise 1:

For this exercise, kneel on both knees and remain upright from the knees up, keeping your back straight. Your knees should be shoulder width apart for this exercise and maintain an erect posture. There will be no pelvic tilting or thrusting for this exercise.

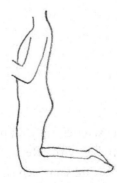

Start slowly. While maintaining an erect posture, contract your PC and hold the contraction for 5 seconds. Follow this with a 5 second rest period. Continue this cycle of contracting, holding, and resting for 30 seconds. Stop and rest for 30 seconds. Then repeat the entire exercise 2 times.

As your muscles get stronger, increase the time you are holding the contraction from 5 seconds to 10 seconds. Follow this with a 5 second rest period. Continue this cycle for 45 seconds. Stop and rest for 45 seconds. Then repeat the entire exercise 2 times.

Continue to increase the time of the contraction until you can hold it for 15 seconds. Follow this with a 5 second rest period. Continue this cycle for 60 seconds. Stop and rest for 60 seconds. Then repeat the entire exercise 2 times.

Exercise 2:

For this exercise, kneel on both knees and remain upright from the knees up, keeping your back straight. Your knees should be shoulder width apart for this exercise and maintain an erect posture.

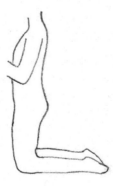

Just as you did in the other exercises, <u>tilt</u> your pelvis forward and backwards at a rate you are comfortable with. Remember tilting does not mean thrusting. While you are tilting your pelvis, contract and hold your PC muscle or the required time.

Start slowly. Tilt your pelvis forward and backward and contract your PC muscle. Hold the contraction for 5 seconds. While you continue tilting your pelvis forward and backwards, rest your PC muscle for 5 seconds. Continue this complete cycle for 30 seconds. Stop everything and rest for 30 seconds. Then repeat 2 times.

As your muscles get stronger, increase the length of the contraction from 5 seconds to 10 seconds. While you continue tilting your pelvis forward and backwards rest your PC muscle for 5 seconds. Continue this complete cycle for 45 seconds. Stop everything and rest for 45 seconds. The repeat 2 times.

Work your way up until you can hold the contraction for 15 seconds. While you continue tilting your pelvis forward and backwards, rest your PC muscle for 5 seconds. Continue this complete cycle for 60 seconds. Stop everything and rest for 60 seconds. Then repeat 2 times.

PART 6

THE PROSTATE

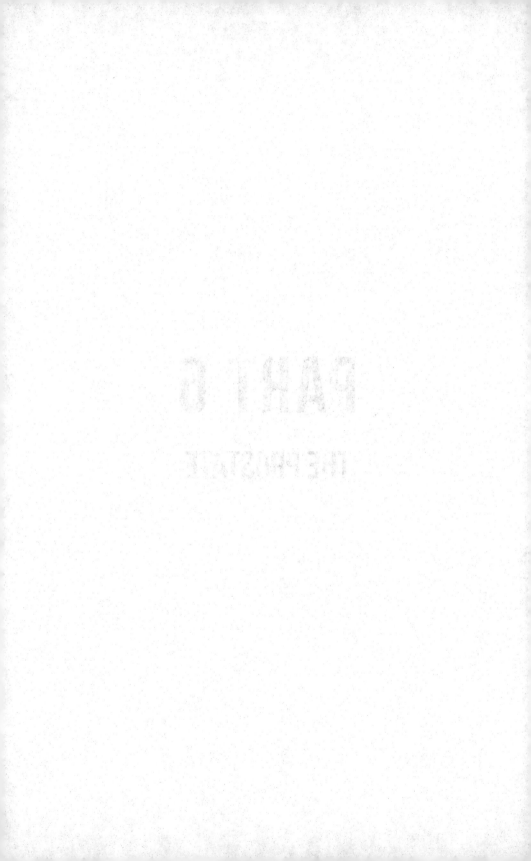

CHAPTER 29

THE PROSTATE

In this chapter we are going to look at the prostate.

The prostate is a small organ (about the size of a walnut) located in front of the rectum and just below the bladder. Its main function is the production of a fluid that together with sperm from the testicles and fluids from other glands make up semen.

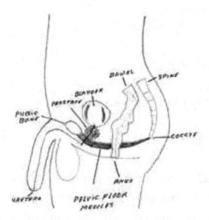

The muscles of the prostate ensure that the semen is forcefully pressed into the urethra (which passes through the prostate). The semen is then expelled outwards during ejaculation.

As men age, the prostate naturally becomes larger. If it becomes too large it can restrict urination by putting pressure on it and causing the urethra to become narrow or completely closed. It can also cause bladder, urinary tract, or kidney problems.

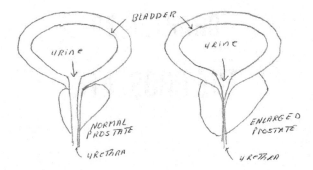

Some of the common signs of a problem with your prostate can include:

A frequent or urgent need to urinate

An increased frequency to urinate at night

Difficulty starting urination

A weak urine stream

The inability to empty your bladder

Dribbling at the end of urination

If you are experiencing any of these symptoms, you should see your doctor. Simply having these symptoms does not mean you have prostate cancer; however, if you are having any of these symptoms you should see your doctor. The severity of these symptoms can vary from person to person, but they tend to worsen over time.

If this doesn't sound bad enough, most of the medications used to treat an enlarged prostate tend to have sexual side effects. Some medications called

Alpha-Blockers have the potential side effect of decreased ejaculation. Instead of semen coming out of the penis it enters the bladder. This is also called a dry orgasm.

This won't hurt you. In fact, you won't be able to tell the difference in the way your orgasm feels. Also, if no ejaculate comes out, your partner may enjoy not having to clean up afterwards. If you are trying to have children, then it becomes a problem. Although technically it is possible for a small amount of sperm to come out with your pre-cum.

Other medications called Alpha Reductase Inhibitors can cause Erectile Dysfunction. A reduced sex drive is a possible side effect of the drug.

I take both medications, so I <u>do</u> know that they can both have these side effects. I can also testify that there is good news waiting for you, even if you do take these medicines.

Let's look at some ways to possibly help avoid prostate problems in the first place. If you check the internet, there are well over 6 million websites to help you "fix" your prostate problems. They will either tell you to take the pills from your doctor, or they will be happy to sell you their pill.

First, do what your doctor tells you to do. Discuss the side effects of any medications with him. Some of the medications are less likely to have sexual side effects. In any case, listen to what he has to say and follow his advice.

If you are having prostate problems, your doctor will either give you a prostate exam or refer you to a specialist who will give you the exam. Yes, he will put on a glove, lubricate his finger, and stick it in your anus.

Then he will rub your prostate to see if it is enlarged or see if there is anything else he can feel inside you. You might just as well do it. It will need to be done.

You can also be a little more proactive. Here are a few things you can do which might help prevent prostate problems.

Of course, the first thing I bring up is Exercise.

Exercising your PC muscle, which is commonly referred to as Kegel exercises, is one of the best things you can naturally do to help. We went over how to do them in chapter 23. Doing the PC muscle flexes should be a part of your regular exercise program.

As well as doing the PC muscle flexes, walking, swimming, jogging (if your ankles and knees are not bothered by this), Yoga, and Qigong are great exercises for helping maintain your prostate health.

Always check with your health care provider before you start any exercise program to make sure you are healthy enough for the exercises.

In our next section, we will be working on some different stretching exercises that will also enhance your sexuality.

Continue to do the exercises that we have already gone through. Keep in mind they will work if you continue to do them.

Don't forget to use your powers of visualization as you work through these chapters and exercises. It really will help.

PART 7
PENIS STRETCHES

CHAPTER 30

THE PURPOSE OF PENIS STRETCHES

The stretching you will do in this section is going to prepare your penis for the next section. For you to understand how and why this works, you need to understand how you get an erection.

Male sexual arousal is a complex process that involves the brain, hormones, emotions, nerves, muscles, and blood vessels. An erection is the result of increased blood flow into your penis.

This Blood flow is (usually) stimulated by sexual thoughts or by direct contact with your penis. In response, your brain sends signals that trigger a hormonal response which allows the penile arteries to open completely.

This allows for increased blood flow through the arteries. The increased blood flow fills the two chambers inside the penis called the Corpus cavernosa (also called Corpora cavernosa) and one chamber on the underside of the penis called the Corpus spongiosum.

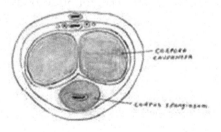

As the chambers fill with blood, they press against the penile veins that allow the blood to flow out. The blood cannot flow out as quickly as it enters, so the penis gets rigid and erect.

An erection ends when the muscles in the penis relax and the blood flows out through the penile veins.

The stretching you do in part 7 will prepare the penis for the new blood you will introduce into it in part 8.

Here is your first stretching exercise.

I will go through the steps of each exercise so you can see exactly how to perform each one. Begin with a warmup.

Start the warmup by squeezing and relaxing your PC muscle. Each squeeze and relaxation is called a flex. Do a set of 30 flexes. At the end of the set, rest for 30 seconds. Continue with 2 more sets, resting for 30 seconds between each set. After the warmup proceed with the stretching:

With one hand grasp your penis just below the head, not so tight that it hurts but have a firm grip. Place the other hand in front of your testicles to hold them in place. Take a deep abdominal breath.

With the hand holding your penis, pull the penis straight out away from your body. Your other hand will hold your testicles in place. When you feel like it has had a sufficient stretch (<u>only you can tell this so go gently</u>) exhale, flatten your stomach, and clench your butt muscles.

Hold this for 30 seconds. Try to hold your breath for the entire 30 seconds if you can. Release your grip and relax for 30 seconds.

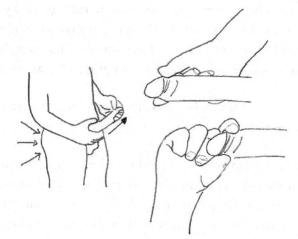

After the 30 second rest, grasp one hand around your penis and with the other hand grasp just above the testicles. Take another deep abdominal breath.

Begin stretching them in opposite directions, again go gently, first stretch with the penis pointing up and the testicles pointing down. At the same time, exhale while flattening your stomach and clenching your butt muscles. When you feel they have stretched far enough (do not overdo it) hold the position for 30 seconds.

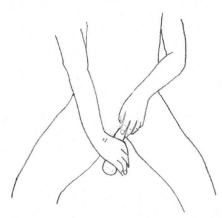

Then release your grip and relax for 30 seconds. After your rest, grasp around your penis and testicles again.

Stretch again only this time pull your penis to the right and your testicles to the left. Don't forget to exhale, flatten your stomach, and clench your butt muscles. After you feel they have stretched far enough, hold that position for 30 seconds. Then release your grip and relax for 30 seconds.

Repeat these steps again only reverse the directions, penis to the left, and testicles to the right.

After your rest, grasp your penis and testicles again. This time you will stretch with the penis pointing down and the testicles pointing up. Don't forget to exhale, flatten your stomach, and clench your butt muscles. Again, when you feel they have stretched enough, hold for 30 seconds. Then release your grip and relax.

In the next chapter, we will continue with some more stretching exercises for your penis.

CHAPTER 31

MORE PENIS STRETCHES

In this chapter we will work on doing more stretches to help enlarge and enhance your penis. Penis Power Stretches are like the testicle stretches from the last chapter but without stretching your testicles.

Continue to use the power of visualization to enhance these exercises.

First the warm-up.

Start with doing one set of squeezing and relaxing your PC muscle which consists of 30 flexes. At the end of the set, rest for 30 seconds. continue with 2 more sets, resting for 30 seconds between each set.

Follow this by warming your hands and penis. Warming the penis will prepare it for this exercise by expanding the tissue and making it more flexible. Do this before every exercise.

Place the palms of your hands together and rub them back and forth to warm them.

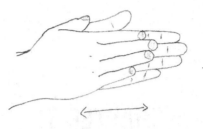

Next hold your penis and testicles between your palms and rub them until they are warm. When they are warm, you will be ready for the penis power stretching.

When you are stretching the penis, you are stretching all parts of the penis. This includes the spongy tissue that fills with blood. When these areas have sufficiently stretched, the penis will extend longer both when it is erect and when it is soft. This is controversial. Some say you can't stretch it, but my wife says it works and it looks to me like it works.

By stretching the flesh and expanding the area that fills with blood, it <u>is</u> possible to enlarge the penis. This will also expand the spongy tissue which will allow more blood to enter it.

In each step of the exercises remember to use your visualization power to <u>vividly</u> see in your mind your penis getting longer and thicker.

First, make sure your penis is in a completely flaccid (soft) state.

Grasp it around the head, but not tight enough to hurt.

Pull the penis out in front of you until you feel it stretch. You will feel this stretch in the middle and at the base. Again, you are not trying to hurt yourself so don't pull too hard.

Hold this stretch for a count of 10.

Rest and try to feel the energy around your sexual organs.

To help get the blood into the stretched area slap your penis against your leg approximately 50 times. Repeat this stretch 3 more times.

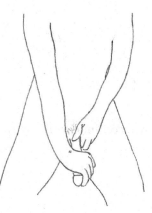

Now grasp the penis again, exhale and flatten your abdomen.

This time, pull your penis to the far left until you feel it stretch on the right side. Hold this stretch for a count of 10. Then release and repeat 3 more times. Again, slap your penis up against your leg approximately 50 times.

Rest and try to mentally "pull" the energy up from your sexual area up to the top of your head. Don't worry if you can't do this yet, it will happen.

For the next step grasp the penis again, exhale and flatten your abdomen. This time, pull your penis to the far right until you feel a stretch on the left side. Hold this stretch for a count of 10. Then release and repeat 3 more times.

Rest and try to mentally pull the energy up from your sexual area to the top of your head. Again, don't worry if you can't do this yet, it will happen with practice.

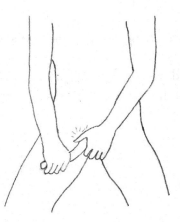

In the next chapter, we will continue with the stretching exercises by doing the Penis Rotations.

CHAPTER 32

PENIS ROTATIONS

In this chapter you will be learning Penis Rotations.

If you are continuing these exercises directly after doing the power stretches and no time has passed for you to cool down, you can skip the warm-up part.

Otherwise, you need to repeat the warm-up.

Start your warm-up by squeezing and relaxing your PC muscle at a steady pace for 30 flexes. At the end of the set, rest for 30 seconds. Continue with 2 more sets, resting for 30 seconds between each set.

Next you will warm your hands and penis. Again, warming the penis will prepare it for the workout by expanding the tissue and making it more flexible. Do this before every exercise.

Place the palms of your hands together and rub them back and forth to warm them. After your hands are warm, place your penis between your hands and rub back and forth until the penis is warm. For this exercise your penis needs to be in a completely "soft" state.

Here is The First Rotation.

Grasp your penis with your hand so your pinkie finger is just behind the head of your penis (your thumb will point toward your stomach) and pull outward until you feel it stretch. Once extended, begin slowly rotating the penis in a circular fashion to your left. Do not twist your penis, simply rotate the entire penis in a circular motion. This will stretch the penis in all areas including the base.

As you rotate the penis, visualize it stretching around the base area. Rotate for 30 rotations and then rest for 30 seconds.

As you rest, gently contract your anus and perineum using your PC muscle. Try to guide, or gently pull the energy from your sexual organs up your back and to the top of your head. Mentally "see" the energy moving along this pathway.

Follow this by slapping your penis against your leg 50 times to allow the new blood to fill the stretched area.

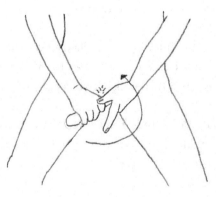

The Second Rotation:

Repeat the steps in the first rotation only this time rotate to your right instead of the left. As you rotate the penis, visualize it stretching around the base area. Rotate for 30 rotations and then rest for 30 seconds.

As you rest, gently contract your anus and perineum using your PC muscle. Try to guide your sexual energy from your sexual organs up your back and to the top of your head. Mentally "see" the energy moving along this pathway.

Follow this by slapping your penis against your leg 50 times.

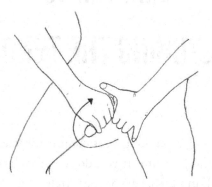

You need to realize the guiding of your sexual energy from your sex organs up to the top of your head is going to take time and practice. But if you take the time and do the practice, the results are going to change your life.

Please don't give up on this. It is very important.

In the next chapter we will continue your stretching exercises by stretching the tendons around your penis and testicles.

CHAPTER 33

STRETCHING THE TENDONS

In this chapter you will be working on stretching the tendons and ligaments around the penis and scrotum. If you do not stretch these, they tend to become tight and shorten. So, part of your stretching exercises will include stretching the tendons and ligaments.

You must do this stretching **gently** because the ligaments and tendons can be damaged. So, **do not rush when doing this exercise**.

As always, I will go over the steps for the exercise.

The first step is to warm your hands by rubbing them together just like we have done in the other exercises. The next step is warming the penis.

Then use your thumb and forefinger to encircle the base of the penis.

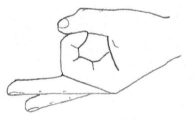

Use your other fingers to encircle and cup your testicles.

Gradually and gently pull your entire groin down toward the tip of your penis as you direct the energy up from your perineum to the 5 major internal organs: the heart, lungs, liver, spleen, and kidneys.

First pull straight down with your hand.

Then pull down and to the left.

Then pull down and to the right.

At the same time as you are doing these downward pulls, flex your PC muscle and pull the energy up from your perineum to your internal organs.

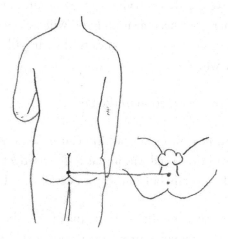

Try to hold this and pull the energy for several seconds. And then release it.

Lastly, pull downwards and in a circular motion for 30 rotations in a clockwise direction. Then reverse direction and rotate for 30 rotations in a counter-clockwise direction.

Now, try to draw your sexual energy upward along your back toward your head.

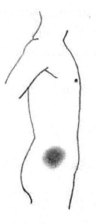

As you can see, we are always trying to move your internal sexual energy. I know this is hard but keep at it and you will succeed in moving it. It's okay to take baby steps when it comes to this. It will happen and it will change your life when it does.

This completes another section of the book.

You have learned how proper breathing can increase your sexual energy. You have learned how visualization has a direct effect on your ability to perform not only sexually but in every aspect of your life.

You have learned how the different organs of your body can affect your sexual energy and how you can enhance your sexual energy by properly massaging these organs.

You have learned about your pelvic floor and how to exercise and strengthen your PC muscle.

You have started the exercises to increase blood flow in your penis.

In the next section you will continue with exercises that will help control your ejaculation.

PART 8

PENIS JELQING

CHAPTER 34

PENIS JELQING

In this chapter I will introduce you to penis jelqing.

In America alone, there are over 30 million men who are impotent or cannot maintain an erection long enough to have sexual intercourse.

A lack of blood circulation in the penis will weaken and shrink the Corpus cavernosa, (the spongy tissue inside the penis). This will also lessen the sensation and feeling during intercourse which will also promote impotence.

If you are having weak erections or times when you can't get an erection, you may have poor blood circulation in your penis and testicles.

Penis jelqing (also called penis milking) will stretch out the tendon-like tissue in the penis making it longer when it is erect as well as when it is soft. You will be forcing blood into the spongy tissue inside the penis. This not only enlarges it but it is also training it to accept more blood flow throughout the entire penis.

Doing this will help you have stronger erections. It will also heighten the sensations and feelings during intercourse. Regular stretching will also ensure a healthier and stronger penis.

A word of caution. If you do this too often or too roughly, you risk making tears in the penis tissue.

When it comes to jelqing, the first thing we need to cover is the use of a lubricant when doing these exercises. Using a lubricant is an absolute must, but not just any lubricant will suffice. If you choose a lubricant that evaporates easily, you will spend a lot of your time reapplying lubricant so you can continue the jelqing.

Baby oil with vitamin E is a good lubricant for exercising. I personally use organic extra virgin coconut oil for my lubricant. I like the smell and it doesn't quickly evaporate.

Next, you will need a mat or towel. This exercise tends to be a little messy. You could drip lubricant on surrounding areas. I always stand on a large towel to prevent this from being a problem.

Now we will start the warm-up.

Start by stretching the penis lightly. Grasp your penis around the head and pull outward. Rotate your penis in a circular motion for 15 rotations, then 15 rotations in the opposite direction. If you feel you need additional rotations for the warm-up, do a few more. But 15 should be enough.

At this point, you can apply the lubricant to your hands. After you apply the lubricant, lightly massage the penis to bring it to a <u>partial</u> erection. You need to have some blood in it for the exercises.

Grasp around the base of the penis shaft with the thumb and forefinger of one hand.

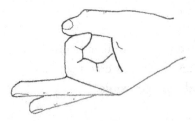

This pressure will retain the blood within the penis, just use enough pressure to keep the blood in the penis.

With your other hand, grasp all the way around the penis. If you grip it too tightly, you risk making the tears. If you grip it too gently, you won't be able to push the blood through the penis properly.

Using the thumb and forefinger of the second hand (the one going around the penis), squeeze all the way around your penis and slide your hand forward slowly. This forces the blood within the penis forward into the erectile tissue and the head. This will take 3 - 5 seconds for each slide.

Visualize your penis lengthening each time you slide down to the head. The blood spaces will expand every time you slide your hand forward.

As your second hand slides forward to the head, the other hand grasps around the base of the shaft keeping the blood trapped inside the penis. Once the sliding hand reaches the head, release it and return it to the base to start another slide. Keep the pressure on the hand in front of your testicles to keep the blood from exiting the penis.

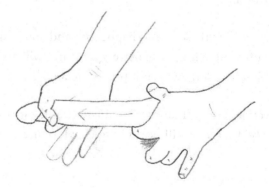

When first starting, some men experience red spots, bumps, or slight bruising on the penis head and surrounding areas. This is not unusual and should subside after the first week of exercise. I experienced this when I first started. Stretching the blood spaces within your penis and the newly increased blood circulation causes this.

If the exercises are painful, stop the exercise. You may be grasping too tightly on the penis. Penis jelqing (milking) is safe if you're not squeezing your penis too hard, too often, or too aggressively.

Being too aggressive can tear tissue or cause damage to the ligaments that connect your penis to your pelvis. Remember from the last chapter, we were stretching them to help with this.

When you are first starting, try to do no more than 100 milkings every other day (this should take less than 2 minutes). I started with a set of 25 followed by a the 15 second warm down. Then I repeated with 4 more sets. Follow the 100 milkings with 15 minutes of warm-down rubbing. Make sure you are also doing at least 100 PC muscle flexes a day.

Continue this every other day for 2 weeks (no more than 4 times in one week. After 2 weeks, you can slowly increase the number of milkings you do up to 600 per day.

As you practice these exercises, you will see your penis getting larger and you will start to notice that it is taking slightly longer for you to reach the point of ejaculation.

The more you visualize these things happening and you "tune in" on the actual feelings of it happening, the more your mind will also believe it is happening. This goes a long way in it becoming a reality.

In the next section, we will start manipulating and moving the sexual energy in your body. These will be exciting chapters and exercises.

PART 9

CIRCULATING YOUR SEXUAL ENERGY

CHAPTER 35

QI AND SEXUAL ENERGY

In this chapter we are going to explore Qi and your sexual energy.

The word Qi (pronounced Chee) has many translations. These include:

Energy

Air

Breath

Lifeforce

Vital essence

Qi has been described as the life-giving force that sustains the entire universe. It is the motion of the atoms in all physical bodies. In short, it is the life-giving sustenance of all the earth.

It is also the life-giving sustenance of your body. Energy must circulate to all parts of your body if you want a healthy body. If the energy in your body is not flowing properly, your body will experience tension, sickness, and disease.

Your sexual energy is the purest form of energy you possess. As a result, it nourishes all parts of your being. This includes your mind, your body, and your spirit. Sexual energy also fuels your emotions. When this energy is in balance it will create a warm, comfortable, glowing energy in your body.

In the chapters to follow, you will start your journey on balancing and moving this energy in your body. I say you will start your journey because this can be a long journey.

Some people find moving their energy to be easy. However, for most people, it is a process that takes time. Like anything worthwhile, it will take some work, but the payoff will be tremendous. Once you successfully learn to move the energy in your body, it will impact your life in ways you cannot imagine.

If you are ready to start this journey, let's go!

First, let's look at the energy circulation system in your body. There are two main channels in your body that circulate the energy.

They are the Governor (Governing) channel which is along your back and the Functional channel (also called the conception or central channel) which runs along the front of your body.

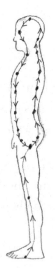

Together the Functional and the Governing channel comprise the Microcosmic Orbit.

The Governor channel begins at the perineum, the point between the genitals and the anus.

This channel runs up through the coccyx (tailbone) and into the spine. From here is goes up the back and through the neck. It then goes over the top of the head and down to a point just behind the eyebrows. It ends at the top of the roof of the mouth just behind the teeth.

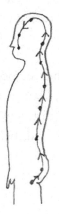

The Functional channel starts at the tip of the tongue and goes down through the neck. It then goes down the chest through your solar plexus and navel. From here it goes past the genitals to the perineum.

To complete the Microcosmic Orbit, we must join these two channels together. Moving the tip of your tongue to the roof of the mouth just behind the front teeth connects the two paths.

Manipulating the energy flow in your body takes time. Do not try to rush this. Everyone's body will respond in its own time.

I find it best to do these exercises with bare feet which will help draw energy up from the earth.

You can control the movement of this energy (Qi) with your mind, or will power if you prefer. This is one reason we have been practicing using the power of visualization.

To begin the process of using the Microcosmic Orbit, concentrate on the point directly behind the navel. (This is the lower Don Tien.) The exact position of the lower Don Tien differs with each person, but generally, it is 1 - 1 ½ inches directly behind and slightly below the navel.

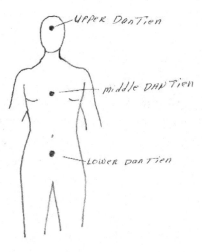

After some practice of concentrating on this area, your navel center will start to feel warm as you concentrate on it. This warm feeling (energy) is what you want to move into the Microcosmic Orbit.

Practice this meditation until you feel the warmness. This is the key to starting everything. It might take 15 minutes, or it may take you a week or more to feel it. You may not feel it for several tries. This is common for most people. Everyone is different, you may not feel it for a while, but it will happen.

As you concentrate, visualize the energy growing in your abdomen. The more you visualize and believe it will happen, the sooner it will happen. Everyone can do this, but it takes time, patience, and dedication to do it.

Most people do not want to put in the time and effort required, so they either don't try or they give up shortly after they start. If they had any idea of the power waiting for them on the other side of the practice, I think they would change their minds.

This is going to change your life if you let it. Once you feel the area behind your naval starting to get warm try to swirl the energy around the navel using your mind.

Do not move on to the next chapter until you can feel the warm energy and are able to move it around your naval. You need to master this first step before you continue with your journey.

When you are ready, we will delve considerably deeper into the Microcosmic Orbit in the rest of the chapters.

CHAPTER 36

THE GOVERNOR CHANNEL

If you are starting this chapter, you were successful in feeling the warm energy behind your naval. You are also able to swirl it around your naval. If you cannot do this, stop, go back to the last chapter, and keep practicing. Then start this chapter.

You will receive a lot of information in this chapter, and you may need to move in steps. You will be able to see where the steps are as you go through the chapter. Make sure you can do each step before you move on to the next one.

Before you continue let me remind you about the use of visualization. I know I have said this many times, but it is so important to the movement of your sexual energy. First, I want you to only imagine moving the energy in your body.

Close your eyes and get a good visual image of your sexual organs as you visualize. Using your mind's eye, visualize a crisp clear picture of the route your energy follows in your Microcosmic Orbit.

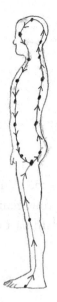

Place the tip of your tongue on the roof of your mouth directly behind your front teeth. Visualize the completed circuit from the roof of your mouth to the tongue.

Next visualize the energy flowing from your perineum up to your tailbone.

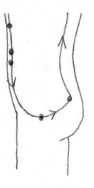

In your mind's eye, see it continue up your back to your neck. Watch it move to the top of your head and start moving down to just behind your eyebrows. See it move to the roof of your mouth and down through your tongue into your neck.

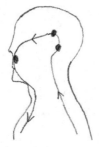

Feel it move down through your chest and solar plexus as it moves into your navel area. Let it move past your genitals and back to the perineum. The more visualization is a standard part of your training, the faster and better the results will be.

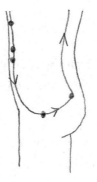

The more you foresee your results and focus on where you want to be, the faster you will get there. Remember, the more real the visualization the easier it will be for your brain to believe it has already happened.

Take the time to visualize this several times before you continue with this chapter.

Now that you have visualized it, let's see if you can start moving your energy. In this chapter we will be working with the Governor channel.

Start by positioning the tip of your tongue at the roof of your mouth, just behind the upper front teeth. Flatten as much of the rest of your tongue up against the roof of your mouth as possible. Leave your tongue in this position for the rest of the practice.

Having your tongue in this position will connect the Governor channel with the Functional channel. Having them connected will allow the energy to flow from one channel to the other.

Next, remove your shoes and socks. Feel the floor, or the ground if you can put your feet on it. Allow the energy from the earth to move up and through your feet.

Think of your feet like tree roots connecting to the earth drawing energy into your body. Allow your mind to pull or guide the energy up from the earth into your feet. This will ground you and keep you connected to the earth.

This may be new to you. So, relax your body and calm your mind. Think of nothing except the earth being a big ball of energy and it is radiating this energy into your feet and legs.

I have used the word allow a few times. You need to give your mind permission to draw or pull energy from the ground. Don't forget. You have not done this before so your mind doesn't know if it should do this or not. Telling yourself that it is okay to do this will have an impact on whether your mind does it or not.

Now, visualize this energy moving into your feet. Let your mind see the energy moving into your feet and then up your legs all the way up to your perineum. After you have given your mind permission to guide the energy up from the earth, you need to visualize it so your mind will <u>see</u> what to do.

Although the feet and legs are not part of the Microcosmic Orbit, allowing the earth energy to move into your feet and up through your legs to the perineum will give you a jump start on moving and controlling your internal sexual energy.

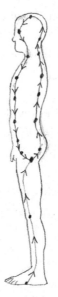

When you feel the energy moving through your feet and legs, focus your attention on the area directly behind and just below the navel. As you focus your attention, visualize the energy building and your navel area starting to warm. Continue this until you can feel the warmness. Now allow your mind to pull, or guide, this warmness down past your genitals to your perineum.

Again, you are giving your mind permission to move this energy. Don't try to rush this. You need time for your mind to focus on the energy and to be able to manipulate it. Give your brain time to understand this. You are directing your mind to do something it has not done before.

If you have not spent time doing meditation, this will be new to you. So, relax your body and calm your mind. Visualize <u>and</u> <u>feel</u> the warm energy moving up to your tailbone.

Your tailbone is the home of your sacral pump. This pump will push the energy from your tailbone up your spine. Flexing your PC muscle tightly and then quickly releasing it help the energy move and activate the sacral pump.

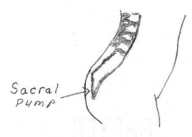

You have not tried to activate this pump before now so it will take a little time for it to respond. If you feel the energy moving up your spine, that is great. If not, try to flex the PC muscle tightly and quickly release it 3 times in a row. Again, you are doing something new with your body. This may take some time, but it <u>is</u> going to happen.

When you feel the energy moving in your spine, allow your mind to pull the energy up your spine toward your head. Feel the warm energy move up through your spine to your neck, to the top of your head, and then to just behind your eyebrows.

At the top of the neck and the back of the head is your cranial pump. This pump works like the sacral pump. It will give the energy a boost and push it into your head and down the Functional channel.

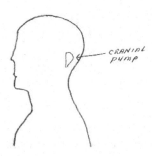

Again, it will help the energy move if you flex your PC muscle tightly and then quickly release the flex to activate the pump. If one flex does not do it, try doing it 3 times in a row.

When you have gotten this far and you can move the energy up to the top of your head, then continue to the next chapter.

CHAPTER 37

THE FUNCTIONAL CHANNEL

If are reading this chapter, you can move the energy from your lower Dan Tien down past your genitals and over to your perineum.

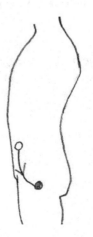

You are also able to move the energy from your perineum to your tailbone and then up your spine. From your spine, you can move the energy up to your head.

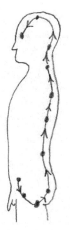

If you can't do this stop, go back, and repeat chapter 36 until you can. If you are unable to move the energy to the top of your head, you can't move it to the Functional channel.

Let's start working with the Functional channel.

First, make sure the tip of your tongue is touching the roof of your mouth just behind the teeth and as much of rest of the tongue as you can, is flat against the roof of your mouth.

Start with allowing the energy from the earth to move into your feet and up your legs. Guide the energy up to your perineum.

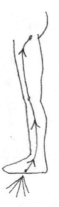

Now, place your attention on the area just behind the naval. Feel the energy start to grow as you feel the warmness of it.

When you feel the energy and the warmness building, direct it down past your genitals and over to the perineum. Let it join the energy flowing up from the earth.

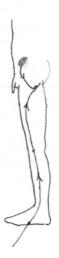

Allow your mind to guide the energy over to your tailbone. Flex your PC muscle and quickly release it and allow the sacral pump to start sending the energy up the spine.

Allow your mind to pull the energy up the spine all the way to the top of the neck and the lower part of the back of your head. Flex your PC muscle and quickly release it and allow the Cranial pump to start sending the energy up to the head.

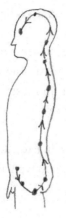

Allow your mind to guide the energy to behind your eyebrows and down to the roof of the mouth. Now, allow your mind to pull the energy through the tip of your tongue.

While you are guiding the energy, visualize the energy moving through the tongue and down through your chest and your solar plexus. Imagine it being a warm beverage flowing through your body.

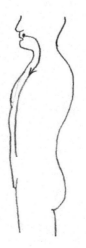

Your sexual energy is the finest and purest energy in your body. And its movement will feel like you are drinking a warm beverage. You will be able to feel the heat going through your body.

Let the energy continue to flow and settle back in the navel area. Once it is in the naval area, it has made one complete cycle.

Practice this meditation as often as time will allow you to practice. Try to do it 3 times a day if possible. Mastering the movement of your energy is not an easy job. But when you do master it, and you will, this will open so many doors for you in life.

Please stay with this until you master it. After you have mastered this, move on to the next chapter where we will talk about your sexual energy and your brain.

CHAPTER 38

SEXUAL ENERGY AND THE BRAIN

In this chapter we will discuss the relationship between your sexual energy and your brain. Let's start at the very beginning. When a fetus is in the mother's womb, for the first 7 to 12 weeks it has no sexual organs.

One could argue that the sex has not been determined at that point so in a way the fetus is both male and female. Although technically, this is not correct. I would, however, say at this point there is a complete balance of yin and yang energy, or the duality in each person.

Your sexual organs have a close connection to the center of your brain, especially the pineal gland. Some consider the pineal gland to be their second sexual organ. You see, sex starts in the brain.

A thought, a desire, or a touch can bring about thoughts of sex. This thought sends signals, in the form of energy, to your sexual organs. Now your sexual energy starts moving.

Your sexual energy cycle has stages. The first stage begins in the brain, at the pituitary and pineal glands, and ends in your sex glands. The second stage returns the energy back to the brain.

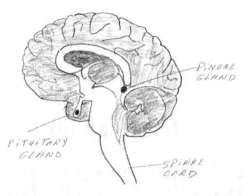

Recycling your sexual energy back to your head will complete the cycle. This will also rejuvenate your brain. You can also use this energy to stimulate your pineal gland and to help open your magical "third eye".

Circulating your sexual energy down to the sacrum (the base of your spine) and back up to the brain will also help increase your memory.

To activate the center of the brain, flex your PC muscle while contracting the eyes, mouth, anus, and prostate gland.

Here is the meditation process.

1) Close your eyes and visualize your sexual organs.

2) Next, visualize the movement of your sexual energy through your microcosmic orbit and let it fill your internal organs.

3) Flex your PC muscle and hold the flex while you mentally pull in on your eyes, mouth, anus, and prostate.

4) Hold this for a few seconds then relax.

Repeat these 3 times.

Every time you do a PC flex, visualize your pineal gland getting bigger.

Here is another method. It is relaxing for your body and I find it easier.

I am referring to spinal breathing. Plan on spending a minimum of 10 minutes doing this meditation. You can do it longer, but plan on at least 10 minutes.

Spinal breathing is a process of bringing your energy up through your spinal column, from your tailbone up to the base of your skull. From here, you guide it to the center of your mind and let it expand throughout your brain to the top of your head.

1) Begin the process, by sitting quietly and putting the tip of the first finger against the tip of the thumb. Do this for each hand.

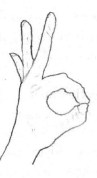

2) Place your hands by your sides with the palms facing upwards.

3) Take a deep breath in through your nose and blow it out your mouth, letting all your frustrations leave the body with the breath. Repeat for 2 or 3 breaths as necessary for you to feel completely relaxed.

4) Bring your attention to the base of the spine and allow the energy to build.

5) As the energy builds, bring it up the spine to the center of your brain and let it continue to expand throughout your head.

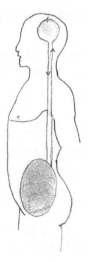

When you breathe in, allow the energy to flow upward to the center and top of the head. When you breathe out, allow the energy to flow back down the spine to the tailbone. Repeat this for several minutes.

Breathe in and let the energy flow up to your head. As you breathe out, let the energy flow down the spine to your tailbone.

Feel a clean white light moving with the energy. The stream of light moves up the spine when you breathe in, and it moves down the spine when you breathe out. Allow the movement of the light and energy to continue for several minutes.

When the light reaches your head, let it expand to fill your head. When it reaches your tailbone, let it expand to fill your pelvic area. The white light expanding in your head will help activate the pineal gland.

Concentrate on moving the energy up and down the spine. Doing this will keep the pathway clear and allow the energy to move freely.

If you perform spinal breathing during sex, when you have an orgasm, it will expand throughout your brain. Not only will you feel euphoric, it may also feel like you are on a mind-expanding drug.

Keep practicing moving the energy in your body. It will change your sex life and it will also enhance every area of the rest of your life.

In the next chapter we will work on Testicle Breathing.

CHAPTER 39

TESTICLE BREATHING

In part 1 you learned the importance of breathing properly. When it comes to accessing and moving your sexual energy, we need to go back to your breathing.

In this chapter you will learn how to do testicle breathing.

If you are not sure you remember the proper breathing exercises, go back, and review part 1. Your breathing is very important so make sure you understand it and you are practicing it.

In part 2 you learned about the power of belief and visualization. You will be using this power to move the sexual energy in your body. If you have not been practicing visualization, go back to part 2 and review the proper way to use your visualization power.

Since you can't physically pick the energy up and move it, you need to use the power of your mind to move it. This is very important, please go back and review visualization if you need to.

Now let's move on to Testicle Breathing.

First, I will go over the exercise and then you can practice it. Do this exercise in a seated position. Use a chair with a firm seat and not a soft cushion.

This is a long exercise, and it will take some time to get proficient at it. If you have been doing your breathing exercises and have been practicing visualization, it will be easier. Take it slowly and don't try to rush through it. The result will be worth all the effort.

1) Sit next to the edge of the chair with your penis and testicles hanging off the edge of the chair.

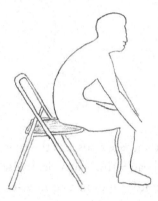

2) Focus your attention on your testicles.

3) Take a deep but gentle breath.

4) Using your mind (and a slight muscular contraction) lift your testicles. This will cause your sexual energy to increase.

5) When your sexual energy starts to increase, use your mind to slowly guide, or pull, the energy to your tailbone.

6) Continue to pull the energy slowly up to your tailbone.

7) Continue to guide the energy up your spine.

8) Gently pull it up to your neck.

9) Continue pulling it until it is all the way into your head.

Repeat these steps 9 more times.

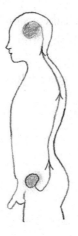

After you have completed these steps and the energy is in your head, spiral the energy inside your head 9 times in a clockwise direction. Then reverse the direction and spiral it 9 times in a counter-clockwise direction.

You have moved the energy up to the top of your head and spiraled it around, now you must complete the cycle.

1) Lift the tip of your tongue to the roof of your mouth just behind your front teeth.

2) Mentally guide the energy down through your tongue.

3) Continue guiding the energy down the front of your body to just behind your navel. This completes the cycle. Leave the energy just behind your navel.

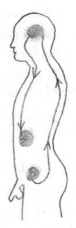

This exercise will strengthen your entire pelvic area as well as bringing sexual energy up to your brain.

Moving energy will have a tremendous impact on your life and your sex life, but it is not going to happen overnight. You may not be able to complete this process on your first few tries.

Getting it up to my brain was the easiest for me. Getting it to move back down the front of my body was the most difficult. But if you practice you will be able to do it.

By now you have been practicing moving your energy quite a bit and you should be able to move it completely through your microcosmic orbit by this time.

I only reminded you that it can be difficult in case you are still having trouble. So, practice doing testicle breathing and we will call this part closed.

This may have been a rough part to get through. Moving energy inside your body can be difficult. If you felt any energy movement in your body, you should consider this a great win. Some gurus spend their entire life learning how to move this energy.

In case you are still having trouble moving the energy in your body, you will be able to move it, but it will take practice. The more you practice and the stronger your visualization, the faster it will happen.

If you continue these exercises and use your visualization powers, you will succeed. You should make working with your energy a part of your daily routine.

This was only the start of moving your energy. There are more advanced classes, but you need to spend time getting the basics down. If you do not have the basic class mastered, you can cause damage to yourself if you try to move into the advanced studies.

Remember, you must make small goals and achieve them and before long you will have achieved the larger goal.

In the next section, we will be discussing foods that can help boost and maintain your sexual energy.

PART 10

DIET

CHAPTER 40

DIET AND YOUR SEX DRIVE

In the next 2 chapters we are going to look at Diet and Your Sex Drive.

Let me ask you a question. Do you exercise or go to the gym and workout? If your answer was yes, or even occasionally, why do you do it?

You will probably say you want to maintain your health and look good.

You may not want to admit it, but the underlying cause most men workout is to improve their chances of having a better sex life or sometimes just improving their chances of having sex.

As you have seen through the other chapters, many things can affect your sex drive and your sexual energy. One we haven't talked much about is your diet.

There are some simple things you can do like skipping the fast-food places and drinking a little less. Doing simple things like that can boost your sex drive.

The trans fats in greasy foods like burgers and fries can drastically reduce the male libido. But many fruits, vegetables, whole grains, and spices can help regulate testosterone and increase your sex drive.

If you need another reason to maintain your weight, one study showed that men with a waist larger than 40" were more likely to have erectile dysfunction than men with a smaller waist. When it comes to being overweight, you need to lose it so you will be ready to use it.

I remember flipping through the channels one day on my TV when Dr. Oz was on and he said something I will never forget. He said, "Men for every 35 pounds you lose you will gain one inch on your penis". Now that is something to think about...

With that in mind, let's go over some specific foods which can <u>hurt</u> your sex drive. Just as there are foods that will enhance your sex drive, there are those which can be <u>detrimental</u> to your sex drive.

Here are some foods you should <u>avoid</u>.

I have already mentioned you should avoid greasy fried foods. Here are some others you need to avoid.

- Processed Foods:

    If you have ever read the labels on your foods, I shouldn't even have to tell you that processed foods are not good for you. They are not good for your heart, your diet, or your sex drive. They tend to be high in trans-fats and sugars. They can reduce blood flow, cause inflammation, lead to you being overweight, and even diabetic.

    All these can have a terrible effect on your sexual energy. According to a Massachusetts study, men who ate a diet of processed and fatty foods showed a spike in erectile dysfunction.

- Overeating:

    The over consumption of any food can lead to weight gain which is the number one sex drive killer, according to the nutritionists at the Metabolic Treatment Center.

- Dairy:

In general, dairy products are rich in saturated fats. These fats get into your bloodstream and increase the likelihood of cardiovascular disease. They can also deposit on the walls of your arteries, which narrows the blood flow.

- Fried Foods:

Fried foods also contain high amounts of fats. These fats can clog arteries and blood vessels which reduce the natural flow of blood into the penis. The penis needs blood flow to achieve and maintain an erection.

When you are eating fried foods, you will also gain weight quicker which could lead to obesity.

- Animal Fats:

Consuming too much animal fat can lead to clogged arteries and blood vessels. Red meat especially causes more adverse consequences. You should limit your consumption of red meat to only once a week. On the other hand, white meats such as chicken or fish have heart-healthy fats and we will discuss this in the next chapter.

Here are some additional things which can have a <u>negative</u> effect on your sex drive.

- Alcohol:

Alcohol may not be a food, but it needs mentioning. The over-consumption of alcohol can influence your sexual health. Alcohol inhibits the production of testosterone, which is responsible for controlling your sexual functions.

Beer contains high levels of estrogen, called the "female" hormone. Consuming high levels of estrogen can throw your hormones out of balance. Not only can this suppress your testosterone production, but high levels of estrogen can also cause the appearance of man-boobs. They are not really breasts, but excess fat stored in your pectorals. It still gives the impression you are growing breasts.

If that is not enough, high levels of estrogen can increase:

Hair loss

Depression

Prostate enlargement

Increased risk of cardiovascular disease

Sexual dysfunction

Exhaustion

Shrinking muscle mass

Reduced growth of penis and testicles

Loss of bone density

Hot flashes

Trouble focusing

Although small amounts of alcohol can reduce your inhibitions and perhaps get you in the mood for sex, over-consumption can have an extremely negative effect on your sex life.

- Smoking:

Let's face it, deep down almost everyone knows that smoking is not good even in the best of times. It contracts and hardens the walls of arteries and blood vessels. Sexual arousal requires good circulation and blood flow, and smoking inhibits the flow of blood.

There is a clear link between erectile dysfunction and cardiovascular health. Doctors and scientists have proven that smoking has a detrimental effect on your cardiovascular health. As an added note, of all the men with reported erectile dysfunction, the smokers outnumbered the nonsmokers by almost 2 to 1.

In the next chapter we will look at some food that can help your sex drive.

CHAPTER 41

GOOD FOODS

In this chapter we will look at some foods that can help increase your sex drive. First on the list are fruits and vegetables. Both fruits and vegetables are powerful when it comes to sexual performance.

- Watermelon:

  Watermelon contains a nutrient called citrulline, which the body converts to arginine. Arginine is an amino acid that boosts nitric oxide levels in the body. You might remember that nitric oxide relaxes the blood vessels in the penis, much the same way Viagra does.

- Beets:

  There have been studies done on consuming beet juice and its effect on nitric oxide levels in the body. In one study, consuming beet-root juice increased nitric oxide levels by 21%.

- Garlic:

  One study showed that aged garlic extract temporarily increased the nitric oxide levels in the blood by 40% within an hour of consumption. It also can help maximize the amount of nitric oxide your body can absorb. Just remember, not everyone appreciates the smell of garlic.

- Meat:

  Meat, poultry, and seafood are excellent sources of CoQ10. Fatty fish, beef, chicken, and pork contain the highest concentration of CoQ10. CoQ10 is a key compound that helps preserve nitric oxide in the body.

- Dark Chocolate:

  Dark chocolate is loaded with flavanols. Research has shown that the flavanols in cocoa can help establish optimal levels of nitric oxide in your body. However, the number of flavanols is (greatly) reduced when processing dark chocolate into milk chocolate. The addition of sugar and fats during processing makes it a high-sugar, unhealthy snack, and foods high in sugar can increase the likelihood of ED.

- Leafy Green Vegetables:

  Leafy green vegetables like spinach, kale, cabbage, arugula, broccoli, brussel sprouts, and chard are packed with nutrients that are converted to nitric oxide. Regular consumption of these can help maintain the levels of nitric oxide in your blood and tissues.

- Citrus Fruits:

  Citrus fruits such as grapefruit, lemons, limes, and oranges are great sources for vitamin C which can also enhance the levels of nitric oxide.

- Pomegranate:

  Pomegranate is high in antioxidants that can protect your cells against damage as well as help preserve nitric oxide.

- Nuts and Seeds:

  Nuts and seeds are high in arginine. Again, arginine is an amino acid that boosts the production of nitric oxide levels in the body.

- Unsweetened Tea:

  Unsweetened tea has an antioxidant called catechin in it and it promotes blood flow all over the body. This is not only good for your sex power but also for your brainpower. It can enhance your memory, mood, and focus.

- Eggs:

  Eggs are rich in vitamins B5 and B6. These vitamins help balance hormone levels and are important for a healthy libido. The yokes, however, are high in cholesterol so not everyone can eat a lot of eggs.

- Oatmeal and other whole grains:

  Oats contain L-arginine which you may remember is an amino acid that enhances the effect nitric oxide has on reducing blood vessel stiffness. Oatmeal is also a natural way to boost testosterone in the bloodstream, which plays a significant role in your sex drive and orgasm strength.

- Oysters:

  It may sound like an old myth, but oysters have more zinc than almost any other food. And it is believed that zinc may enhance your libido by helping with testosterone production. Zinc is also crucial to healthy sperm production and blood circulation.

- Beans:

  While beans may not be your first choice before a night of sex, they are packed full of cholesterol-lowering soluble fiber. Red kidney beans also have more than 6,000 disease-fighting antioxidants. Navy beans are rich in potassium which regulates blood pressure and heart contractions.

So, the bottom line is: If you want to have a healthy sex drive, skip the fast foods and processed foods. Instead, eat a healthy diet of fruits and vegetables, specifically, leafy green vegetables, fish, poultry, pork, and small amounts of red meats.

You have reached the end of the book, so what's next?

First and foremost: Don't stop doing the exercises and meditations you have learned. Continue them daily, or at least every other day. Continue to use your power of visualization and mindset to achieve your goals. If your brain believes something is real, it will make it a reality.

Also, the things you are doing in this book have been practiced for thousands of years by the Chinese and they do work, but you must give it time and keep at it. I know these methods work. They have worked in my life, and they will work in yours. Just give it the time it needs to become a reality.

Next, get some exercise. Exercise is also key to staying in shape sexually. Qigong is an excellent way to stay in shape and increase your sexual energy.

Watch your diet. Being overweight is one of the leading causes of erectile dysfunction.

And remember, if you believe you can do it, you are right.

If you believe you cannot do it, you are right.

It all comes down to what you <u>choose</u> to believe.

ABOUT THE AUTHOR

Having suffered the effects of ED and learning first hand the devastation, self doubt, and the feelings of being less of a man than he was before, Bill delved deeply into the ancient art of restoring his sexual youth. Now, he wants to share his triumph with you and teach you how to Conquer YOUR Erectile Dysfunction.

Printed in the United States
by Baker & Taylor Publisher Services